Think Yourself to Health, Wealth & Happiness

Titles by Joseph Murphy

THE POWER OF YOUR SUBCONSCIOUS MIND

THE MIRACLE OF MIND DYNAMICS

YOUR INFINITE POWER TO BE RICH

SECRETS OF THE I CHING

THE AMAZING LAWS OF COSMIC MIND POWER

THINK YOURSELF RICH

THINK YOURSELF TO HEALTH, WEALTH & HAPPINESS

PUTTING THE POWER OF YOUR SUBCONSCIOUS MIND TO WORK

Think Yourself to Health, Wealth & Happiness

The Best of Dr. Joseph Murphy's Cosmic Wisdom

Joseph Murphy, Ph.D., D.D.
Compiled and edited by David H. Morgan

PRENTICE HALL PRESS

PRENTICE HALL PRESS
Published by the Penguin Group
Penguin Group (USA) Inc.
375 Hudson Street, New York, New York 10014, USA
Penguin Group (Canada), 90 Eglinton Avenue East, Suite 700, Toronto, Ontario M4P 2Y3, Canada
(a division of Pearson Penguin Canada Inc.)
Penguin Books Ltd., 80 Strand, London WC2R 0RL, England
Penguin Group Ireland, 25 St. Stephen's Green, Dublin 2, Ireland (a division of Penguin Books Ltd.)
Penguin Group (Australia), 250 Camberwell Road, Camberwell, Victoria 3124, Australia
(a division of Pearson Australia Group Pty. Ltd.)
Penguin Books India Pvt. Ltd., 11 Community Centre, Panchsheel Park, New Delhi—110 017, India
Penguin Group (NZ), 67 Apollo Drive, Rosedale, North Shore 0632, New Zealand
(a division of Pearson New Zealand Ltd.)
Penguin Books (South Africa) (Pty.) Ltd., 24 Sturdee Avenue, Rosebank, Johannesburg 2196, South Africa

Penguin Books Ltd., Registered Offices: 80 Strand, London WC2R 0RL, England

While the author has made every effort to provide accurate telephone numbers and Internet addresses at the time of publication, neither the publisher nor the author assumes any responsibility for errors, or for changes that occur after publication. Further, the publisher does not have any control over and does not assume any responsibility for author or third-party websites or their content.

First edition: November 2002

Library of Congress Cataloging-in-Publication Data

Murphy, Joseph, 1898–1981.
    Think yourself to health, wealth and happiness : the best of Joseph Murphy's cosmic wisdom / Joseph Murphy ; compiled and edited by David H. Morgan.
        p. cm.
    ISBN 978-0-7352-0363-1
    1. New Thought. I. Morgan, David H. (David Huw), 1942– II. Title.
    BF639.M839 2002
    299'.93—dc21   2002021953

146122990

Intuition

The Supreme Intelligence,
or Life Principle in your subconscious,
is always knocking at the door of your heart.

Open the door to your heart and listen.

Contents

Part I
THE GREAT LAWS OF THE SUBCONSCIOUS MIND

Chapter 1
Understanding the Laws of the Subconscious

Chapter 2
The Dynamic Power of Your Thoughts and Affirmations

Part II
ENRICH YOUR LIFE WITH THE UNLIMITED POWER OF YOUR SUBCONSCIOUS MIND

Chapter 11
Your Unlimited Power to Overcome Worry and Fear

Chapter 12
Your Unlimited Power to Overcome Negative Thinking

Chapter 13
Your Unlimited Power to Achieve Prosperity

Acknowledgments

I would like to thank JMW Group, Inc., for giving me the opportunity to work on this book. It is always nice to have work, to have something to do. It is especially nice when what you do inspires and enriches you, as the writings of Joseph Murphy have done for me.

In particular, I would like to thank Pete Allen and Sara Castle, of JMW Group, Inc, for their support and infinite patience. They will smile when they read that, no doubt think that "infinite" falls far short of describing the degree of patience they were required to exercise. I don't know of a word that speaks of a greater quantity. If I did, I would use it, for they have given it. Perhaps where I'm falling short, then, is not in the word *infinite*, but in the word *patience*. Perhaps I should instead have used *forbearance*. So I will revise my gratitude: I would like to thank Pete Allen and Sara Castle for their infinite forbearance.

My thanks to production editor Mariann Hutlak, for her generosity of time and her guidance in seeing to it that a manuscript became a book.

And I would be remiss if I excluded my cat Toby. He has had to endure months of regrettable neglect. But always, he came to me, giving his affection, seeking mine. Often, he received instead my ill temper, my impatience, as he uncannily entered my office at just those moments when I was struggling for a word or concept or the order of things. In the end, however, he won me over, reminding me in the process of what I think is perhaps one of Joseph Murphy's most profound teachings: (which you'll find in his chapter "Forgiveness"): "Without love in our hearts, we stumble and fall."

What This Book Can Do for You

*T*hrough the words you will read, you will discover the limitless power within you to create the life of prosperity and harmony you desire. You will learn to tune in to the infinite intelligence and power within you.

Think Yourself to Health, Wealth & Happiness contains the keys to transforming your life. Bringing together the highlights of Joseph Murphy's lifetime of teachings about the power of the subconscious mind, this book will help you learn the rules, techniques, and principles for using the power of your subconscious to bring forth health, happiness, prosperity, and all that you desire in your life.

To reap the greatest benefit from this book, start by reading all of Part I, "The Great Laws of the Subconscious Mind," in order to acquire an understanding of the basic principles of the power of the subconscious mind. A firm grasp of these is essential. Part II, "Enrich Your Life with the Unlimited Power of Your Subconscious Mind," will guide you in applying the laws of the subconscious to specific areas of your life that you seek to change or enhance. As you read Part II, allow yourself to stay with each chapter for a while. Take time to reflect on it and understand how it addresses your current needs. Allow the teachings of the chapter to become a part of your subconscious. Then move on to another chapter.

Once you have concluded your initial reading of the book, keep it on hand as a companion that you can turn to whenever you want to enrich an area of your life or are facing a difficulty of any kind. For example, if you want to know more about the miraculous power of prayer and how you can benefit from it, you can turn to Chapter 4; if you're finding it difficult to forgive, you can turn to Chapter 5; if needless worry and fear are holding you back, Chapter 11 will teach you to find peace; and if you are seeking more fulfilling relationships, Chapter 17 will guide you.

Joseph Murphy dedicated his life to understanding the laws of the subconscious mind and to teaching others—in simple, down-to-earth terms—how to translate this understanding into practical techniques that can be applied for the betterment of everyday life. In these pages, you will find invaluable knowledge culled from Murphy's teachings and particularly chosen for inclusion here because of their keenness of insight and practical benefits. You will read about real people and how they used the laws of the subconscious to bring desired changes into their life. You will discover techniques that you can apply to strengthen the power of your subconscious and use to achieve all your aspirations and you will learn the key principles to remember and apply in your daily life. Whatever enrichment or transformation your desire, *Think Yourself to Health, Wealth & Happiness* will help you attain it.

Editor's Preface

Think Yourself to Health, Wealth & Happiness

The Best of Joseph Murphy's Cosmic Wisdom

Part I

THE GREAT LAWS OF THE
SUBCONSCIOUS MIND

1 Understanding the Laws of the Subconscious

What you can conceive, you can achieve through the
wisdom and power of your subconscious mind.

■

Your subconscious is part of mind, which operates in accordance with psychological laws, and part of Mind, which operates in accordance with spiritual laws. This is not to say that the subconscious is two minds. It is one mind that can have two distinct ways of operating. To truly understand then, the workings, and most importantly the *power* of your subconscious, it is important—indeed necessary—that we discuss and know well its two aspects, or operations, separately.

THE SUBCONSCIOUS AS HABIT–MIND

It often appears as though we are living in two worlds: one external and the other internal; one visible and the other invisible; one objective and the other subjective.

The external (visible, objective) world enters you through your five senses and is shared by everyone. Your internal (invisible, subjective) world of thoughts, feelings, imagination, sensations, beliefs, and reactions belongs to you alone.

Suppose, for example, that you are invited to a banquet. Everything that you see, hear, taste, smell, and touch is of the external world, the world revealed by your five senses. All that you think, feel, like, and dislike belongs to your inner world. In one sense, it could be said that you are attending two banquets: the one of your sensory experiences and the one of your subjective experiences. In the end, though, there is only one banquet: the one of your subjective experience. Even your sensory experiences would mean nothing if it weren't for your subjective experiences that tell you that you like this and don't like that, enjoy this and don't enjoy that, want this and don't want that.

Ask yourself, "In which world do I do my living? Do I live in the world that is revealed by my five senses, or in the inner world?"

In truth, it is in the inner world that you live all the time. Whether you are acting so consciously or not, it is in this world where you hold your truest existence. This is the world of your subconscious. This is where you feel. This is the world you want to consciously honor in order to have the life you want.

The law of your mind is this: You will get a reaction or response from your subconscious mind according to the nature of the thought or idea you hold in your conscious mind.

The terms generally used to distinguish the two functions of your mind are objective and subjective mind, conscious and subconscious mind, waking and sleeping mind, surface self and deep self, voluntary mind and involuntary mind, male and female—

among others. I use the terms *conscious* and *unconscious* to represent this dual nature of your mind.

It is important to remember, however, that these are not two minds. They are merely two spheres of activity within one mind. *You have only one mind, which possesses two distinctive characteristics, two levels.*

The functions of these two spheres of mind are essentially unlike. Each is endowed with separate and distinct attributes and powers.

The five-sense mind, the conscious mind, is the mind that thinks from the standpoint of circumstance, conditions, and environment, but it is within your subconscious mind that you will find the cause for every effect. The conditions, circumstances, and environment of your life are not the cause of your life—they are the effects.

Your conscious mind has the thought of expectancy; your deeper mind has the "know-how" of accomplishment. Consider this parable of the conscious and subconscious minds.

The captain of a ship directs the ship and signals orders to those in the engine room who control all the boilers, instruments, gauges, and so on. The workers in the engine room do not know where they are going; they follow orders. They would go on the rocks if the person on the bridge issued faulty or wrong instructions. The captain issues orders that are automatically obeyed. Those in the engine room do not give their input; they simply carry out orders.

Our subconscious convictions and beliefs dictate and control all our conscious actions.

The subconscious acts by law. The law that may now hold you in bondage can also be the law that can free you. A negative habit that binds you can be transformed into a positive habit that frees you, through the repetition and the abiding conviction of your desired action in your conscious mind.

Habits, in other words, are formed by repeating certain thought patterns or actions over and over again until they establish patterns in the subconscious mind, where they grow until they reach the point of saturation. Impressions are made in the subconscious by repetition, faith, and expectancy. Whatever is repeated by you over and over again becomes an established habit pattern and is in control.

Through the act of repetition and conviction, your newly desired conscious *will* for yourself can become your *subconscious* will for yourself.

Your subconscious mind works twenty-four hours a day, pouring all the fruit of your habitual thinking into your life.

The law of the subconscious mind does not act differently for the rich or the poor, the good or the wicked. It produces unerringly what it is presented. If you hold up a horrible painting in front of a mirror, the mirror will reflect exactly the picture held before it. The subconscious mind is a mirror for the king and the beggar alike: It always reflects accurately the contents of your mentality.

Just as a doctor has confidence when he or she begins to operate, because the doctor knows surgery, anatomy, physiology, and other basic sciences dealing with the human body, you can, by comparable study and application, develop confidence in the principles of the two functions of your mind—namely the conscious and subconscious. You can learn that the subconscious mind responds to your habitual thinking, and that by carefully choosing your thoughts, you can choose your reactions and responses to life, thus creating the life you want.

Your conscious mind is the reasoning, thinking mind. You make all your decisions with your conscious mind. Your subconscious mind is the seat of your emotions and is the creative mind.

Your conscious mind chooses, but it does not create. Your subconscious is the creative power within you. By the combined operations of your subconscious and conscious minds, you truly become the sum total of your conscious choices.

If you say to your subconscious, "Wake me up at six o'clock," you will awaken exactly at the time specified. It never fails. The subconscious is a source of omnipotent power.

If you pay keen attention to the actions and behaviors of your conscious life and the ideas that well up in your conscious mind, you will find that your subconscious mind is attempting to keep you informed of things transpiring on the subjective plane of your life. It is always trying to support you. The law of life is self-preservation.

You have free will in the choice of the idea, desire, or concept you entertain. In that sense, you have freedom. Thereafter, however, once you mentally accept an idea as living reality, all your steps are then controlled by the subconscious mind, which operates according to the law of compulsion. The beliefs and assumptions that have become embedded in your subconscious dictate, control, and govern all your conscious actions.

Only through the conscious choice of the prayer to change your subconscious beliefs for the better can you alter the movement of the law of compulsion in your life.

The wisdom of your deeper mind is always using you. Practice using the wisdom of your deeper mind until it begins to use you in such a manner that all your ways are pleasant and all your paths are peace.

The law of the subconscious is the universal and natural principle of action and reaction: Whatever you impress on your subconscious mind by your conscious mind will be expressed, that is, carried out in your life.

As Ralph Waldo Emerson said: "There is no thought in my mind but it quickly tends to convert itself into a power and organizes a huge instrumentality of means."

◼

*W*hatsoever a man soweth, that shall he also reap
(Galatians 6:7)

This refers to the action of our thoughts. We *sow* thoughts
when we believe them wholeheartedly.

Our subconscious minds are like the soil. They will grow
whatever type of seed we plant in the gardens of our minds, and
that is what we will reap.

◼

Your subconscious accepts and brings into reality the dominant of two ideas, feelings, and images. It is your dominant
thoughts, feelings, and images that control all phases of your life.

◼

In thinking about your subconscious mind, remember that it
operates deductively. It brings to a logical, sequential conclusion
the nature of the thoughts, feelings, or pictures you hold in your
conscious mind.

◼

Your conscious mind is referred to as your objective mind
because it deals with outward objects; it takes cognizance of the
objective world. It is your guide and director in your contact with
your environment. It learns through observation, experience, and
education—acquiring knowledge through your five senses.

Your subconscious mind is referred to as your subjective mind because it takes cognizance of its environment by means independent of the five senses. It perceives by intuition. It is the seat of your emotions and the storehouse of memory.

The only thing necessary for you to do is to get your subconscious mind to accept your idea, and the law of your own subconscious mind will bring it forth. You give the command or decree, and your subconscious will faithfully reproduce the idea impressed upon it.

Innumerable experiments by psychologists and others on persons in the hypnotic state have shown that the subconscious mind is incapable of making decisions and comparisons that are necessary for a reasoning process. These experiments have shown repeatedly that your subconscious mind will accept any suggestion, however false. Having once accepted any suggestion, it responds according to the nature of the suggestion given.

The subconscious mind works by the association of ideas and uses every bit of knowledge that you have gathered in your lifetime to bring about its purpose. Once the subconscious mind accepts an idea, it begins to execute it; in accordance with the law of compulsion, it works for good and bad ideas alike. You will get a reaction or response from your subconscious mind according to the nature of the thought or idea you hold in your conscious mind: If you think good, good will follow; if you think evil, evil will follow. It does not reason things out the way your conscious mind does, and it does not argue with you controversially. It does not engage in proving whether your thoughts are good or bad, true or false, but accepts what is impressed upon it or what you consciously believe and responds accordingly. Whatever you claim mentally and feel as true, your subconscious mind will accept and bring forth into your experience. If you consciously assume something as true, even though it may be false, your subconscious mind will accept it as true, proceeding to bring about the results which must necessarily follow, because you consciously assumed them to be true.

The law of the subconscious is always impartial, impersonal, and neutral. Your subconscious mind is amoral and impersonal, it is neither compassionate nor vindictive; it has no morality. Morality depends on your motivation and how you use the law of mind.

Your desires are good or bad depending on the nature of the desire itself. Your thought carries its own reward. Desire good, and by the immutable law of your subconscious mind, good follows.

This is the way your mind works.

It is neither more nor less than the law of cause and effect, which is a universal and impersonal law.

We are creatures of habit. If we repeat a thought or act over a period of time, instilling it into our subconscious minds, we will be under the compulsion of a habit, because habit is the function of our subconscious minds. We learned to swim, ride a bicycle, dance, and drive a car by consciously doing these things over and over again until they established tracks in our subconscious minds. Then, the automatic habit action of our subconscious minds took over, resulting in the performance of actions that we now call "second nature."

We are free to choose our thoughts—noble or ignoble. We

are free to choose a good habit or a bad habit. Once we choose, our lives are then lives of either good habits or bad habits.

※

You are always writing the book of your life, because your thoughts become your experiences.

What you write on the inside, you will experience on the outside. If something is written on your subconscious mind, your subconscious mind will move heaven and earth to bring it to pass, and you will experience it in your life as the objective manifestation of circumstances, conditions, and events. Impress your subconscious with right ideas and constructive thoughts, for as Emerson said, "Man is what he thinks all day long."

※

The reason we experience so much personal suffering and pain is that we do not understand the interaction between the conscious and subconscious minds. The subconscious mind is a law: It arranges all of the conscious thoughts we deposit into it into a complex pattern. These patterns become the cause of all our ills, as well as the cause of our triumphant achievements.

Psychiatrists and psychologists delving and probing into our deeper minds have demonstrated that we are not aware of these inner patterns. Not having placed them there knowingly, many of us assume that we don't even have them. Then we establish alibis and excuses of all kinds to justify ourselves and the behaviors we manifest.

Unless otherwise checked, the conscious mind, with its evidence based on the five senses and outer appearances, often interferes with the innate, life-giving movement of the subconscious. Then fear, false beliefs, and negative patterns are made to register in your subconscious mind, and there is no other course open to the subconscious mind except to act on these suggestions and bring them into your life, resulting in your suffering and pain.

When the principles of the conscious and subconscious minds work in accord and synchronously toward harmony, you bring yourself a life of happiness and peace.

***

You can look upon your mind as being like an iceberg, 90 percent of which is subconscious and "below water."

Your subconscious is the major operator of your life; its beliefs dictate, control, and manipulate all your conscious actions. More than 90 percent of your mental life, therefore, is subconscious. Those who fail to understand the workings of this incredible power live within very narrow limits.

***

Your subconscious is amenable to the suggestions of your conscious mind just as well as the suggestions of another's, if their suggestions are accepted as true by your conscious mind. You can always reject the suggestions of others, though, by thinking on whatsoever things are true, lovely, and of good report.

***

Although your subconscious mind is all-wise and knows all the answers to all questions, it does not argue with you or talk back to you. It does not say, "You must not impress me with that thought." It accepts the ideas—true or false—given it by your conscious mind, working deductively to bring your thoughts into your life with unwavering focus and accuracy.

Everything you experience is due to the law of mind. By dwelling on the idea of increased good, and by nourishing it and sustaining it, you draw more of the riches of life to yourself. On the other hand, if you think only of decrease, lack, and limitation, you magnify your loss.

The law of your subconscious is to increase any idea implanted in it.

THE SUBCONSCIOUS AS UNIVERSAL MIND

Your subconscious mind is one with Infinite Intelligence and Boundless Wisdom. It is fed by hidden springs, and is called the Law of Life. Your subconscious mind is also a manifestation of Universal Mind.

There is a Power in you that has never been fully released. God dwells in you rather than operating or influencing you from without. The Power that moves the world and governs the galaxies in space, in other words, is *within you*. You have, then, through your subconscious mind, the infallible power to direct the Cosmic Power that created the universe! This Power stands always at your beck and call and obeys your decrees and beliefs. It is your obedient servant and awaits only your use and direction. It is inexhaustible, eternal, and infinite.

Surrender to this Power and let its beneficent, healing balm flow through your body, business, home, life, and finances. Once you get the knack of directing it, you will find that it will heal your ailing body, ailing pocketbook, ailing human relationships, and ailing heart. It is impossible for you to exhaust the infinite riches of the Universal Mind. Your subconscious then, as a manifestation of Universal Mind, is your most powerful friend and ally.

Your subconscious is sometimes referred to as the soul.

Your subconscious mind is the source of your ideals, aspirations, and altruistic urges.

Your mind is a part of the One Universal Mind: God. When you use your mind in the right way, you gain a response from this Deeper Mind.

There is in all of nature a law of action and reaction, or cause and effect. In mental activity, thought is the action, and the response of the subconscious mind is the reaction.

If you set up resistance in your mind to the flow of Life through you, you're going to get a reaction: Emotional congestion will get snarled up in your subconscious mind and cause all kinds of negative conditions in your life.

That is why it's of such importance to harmonize your conscious thoughts with what you know to be the operation of the subconscious mind: *Be sure that you think on whatsoever things are true, whatsoever things are honest, whatsoever things are just, whatsoever things are pure; whatsoever things are lovely, whatsoever things are of good report, if there be any virtue, and if there be any praise, think on these things.* (Philippians 4:8)

There is a Power and Intelligence within you that far transcends your intellect.

You are living in a fathomless sea of infinite riches. Within your subconscious depths lie the Infinite Wisdom, Infinite Power, and Infinite Supply of all that is necessary, waiting for development and expression. The Infinite Intelligence within your subconscious mind can reveal to you everything you need to know at every moment of time and point of space, provided you are open-minded and receptive. Whatever you desire, there is a power that can fulfill that desire for you; there is an answer to every problem.

The master secret of the ages, then, is not the secret of atomic energy, thermonuclear energy, or interplanetary travel. The secret is that there is a marvelous, miracle-working power found in your own subconscious mind.

You can bring into your life more power, wealth, health, and happiness by learning to contact and release the hidden power of your subconscious mind. You need not acquire this power: you already possess it. But you must learn how to use it; you must understand it, so that you can apply it in all departments of your life.

Begin to control your thought processes and you will be able to apply the Power of your subconscious to any problem, as you will actually be consciously cooperating with the Infinite Power and Omnipotent Law that governs all things.

It is your right to discover your inner world of Power, Light, Love, and Beauty. Then you will discover the greatest truth: The law of your subconscious, when properly used, cannot fail you.

▓

The other day in a restaurant I heard a man say to his companion that sometime, he would hit the jackpot and make his mark in the world. The other replied, "I hope someday I will get a healing for my arthritis." They were postponing their good, and looking to the future for its fulfillment.

All the powers of the Cosmic Mind are *within you now*. Most people are *waiting* for something good to happen in their lives, instead of realizing that God is the Eternal Now. They are constantly saying that "some day" they will be happy, prosperous, and successful.

Wealth is available now; it is a thought-image in your mind. Why wait for it?

Strength is now. Call on the infinite Power of God within you, and this Power will respond, energizing, vitalizing, and renewing your whole being.

Love is now. Know and believe that God's love envelops and saturates your mind and body, and that this Divine love will be filtered through and made manifest in all phases of your life.

Guidance is now. Infinite Intelligence within you knows the answer, and responds to the nature of your request.

Peace is now. Fulfillment is now.

Healing is now. The Infinite Presence that made you is flowing through you now: transforming, healing, and restoring every atom of your being.

Claim your good now. Now is the time.

Remember, you do not create anything; all you do is give form and expression to that which always was, now is, and ever shall be.

❖

The Bible says, *"Ask, and it shall be given you; seek, and ye shall find; knock, and it shall be opened unto you: For everyone that asketh receiveth: and he that seeketh findeth; and to him that knocketh it shall be opened. Or what man is there of you, whom if his son ask bread, will he give him a stone? Or if he ask a fish, will he give him a serpent?"* (Matthew 7:7–10)

Here the Bible tells you to ask, seek, and knock and you will receive a response from your subconscious mind, whose nature is responsiveness. Become enthusiastic, and feel and know that there is a solution to every problem, a way out of every dilemma, and that when you ask for bread, you will not get a stone, but rather the embodiment of your request.

There are no incurable conditions, for with God all things are possible.

❖

Your subconscious mind is such a powerful force, because within your subconscious mind is the Divine Presence. You can call this Presence your Higher Self, the Superconscious, the I Am, or the Christ in you, the hope of Glory, Inner Wisdom, Universal Mind, the Life Principle, Subliminal Mind, or Superconscious Mind. All these terms mean the same thing.

All you need to know is that there is an Infinite Wisdom and Intelligence within you that far transcends your intellect or your five senses—and that it always responds to your recognition, faith, and expectancy.

▓

The subconscious uses all its mighty resources to begin manifesting your idea in your life; to that end, it mobilizes all the mental and spiritual laws of your deeper mind. What is of the utmost importance to remember is that the principle of the subconscious works for good or bad ideas. Consequently, if you use it negatively, it brings trouble, failure, and confusion. When you use it constructively, it brings guidance, freedom, and peace of mind. *For whatsoever a man soweth, that shall he also reap.* (Galatians 6:7)

▓

What you decide to be true with your conscious mind, you will experience with your subconscious mind. It is of the utmost importance, therefore, to begin now to believe, claim, feel, and know that God is guiding you in all ways; that Divine right action governs you at all times; that God is prospering you in all ways; and that you are inspired from On High. As you accept these truths with your conscious mind, your subconscious will bring them to pass, and you will discover that all your ways are pleasantness and all your paths are peace.

▓

We cannot analyze the mind under a microscope, nor can we see it, but like any other force, we can pay attention to how it works. As we study the operations of the mind, its ways cease to seem magical, but they remain marvelous.

Study the ways of your mind, and you will discover a wondrous, hidden power that will raise you up and set you on the high road to happiness, freedom, and peace of mind. Wonders will happen in your life.

░

Many people constantly say that there is no way to solve their problems, that their situations are hopeless. Such an attitude is the result of, and results in, spiritual blindness.

We begin to see spiritually—which is the same as mentally, because the mind is Spirit—when we gain a new understanding of our mental powers and develop a conscious awareness that the Wisdom and Intelligence in our subconscious can solve all our problems.

░

To bring about an answer to your concern, your subconscious mind draws on the Infinite Power, Energy, and Wisdom within you. It lines up all the laws of nature to get its way. Sometimes it brings about an immediate solution to your difficulties, but at other times it may take days, weeks, or longer.

I once told a man, "If you use your subconscious mind in the right way, it will provide you with what you need."

"How? Please, tell me," he begged.

"You're not to wonder how, when, or where," I replied. "Don't wonder about the source. The subconscious has ways you know not of. Its ways are past finding out."

░

When you are seeking an answer to a problem, your subconscious will respond, but it expects you to have a firm conviction in your conscious mind. This does not mean that you must already know the answer or that you can't ask your subconscious about conflicting concerns you're having. It means that you must acknowledge that the answer *is* in your subconscious mind. It means that you must unhesitatingly accept that the solution lies within the problem, that the answer is in every question, and that Infinite Intelligence within your subconscious mind knows all and sees all, has the answer, and is revealing it to you now. This mental attitude that the Creative Intelligence is bringing about a happy solution will enable you to find the answer.

You can't, however, request an answer from your subconscious while consciously thinking, "I don't think there is any way out; I am all mixed up and confused; why don't I get an answer?" By doing that, you would be neutralizing your prayer.

Harmonize the conscious and subconscious mind. Turn over your request to your subconscious mind with the conscious conviction that it has the know-how of accomplishment and that it will respond to you according to the nature of your request.

When the conscious and subconscious minds cooperate, the idea or desire implanted in the subconscious mind is always realized.

It is of great importance to realize that your subconscious mind is always working. It never sleeps; it never rests. It is always on the job. Its Power is enormous. It is the source of Power and Wisdom that places you in touch with the Omnipotence and the Power that moves the world, that guides the planets in their course, and that causes the sun to shine. It is active night and day, whether you act upon it or not.

The reason you often cannot argue rationally in defense of your profoundest convictions is that they do not come from your conscious, reasoning mind; they come from your subconscious mind.

▓

Your subconscious speaks to you in intuitions, impulses, hunches, intimations, urges, and ideas, and it is always telling you to rise, transcend, grow, advance, and move forward to greater heights.

▓

The urge to love, to save the lives of others, to act altruistically, to suspend concern for your own life in times of crisis, comes from the depths of your subconscious, because the law of the subconscious is the law of God, and the law of God is the law of right action.

▓

Your subconscious will speak lofty and wise sayings through you that your conscious mind knows nothing about. Throughout history, great artists, musicians, poets, speakers, and writers have known this and have tuned in to their subconscious powers and become inspired.

Robert Louis Stevenson used to charge his subconscious with the task of evolving stories for him while he slept. He was accustomed to asking his subconscious to give him a good, marketable thriller when his bank account was low. Stevenson said the intelligence of his deeper mind gave him the story piece by piece, like a serial.

Mark Twain confided to the world on many occasions that he never worked in his life. All his humor and all his great writings were due to the fact that he tapped the inexhaustible reservoir of his subconscious mind.

Self-preservation is the first law of life. The Infinite Intelligence of your subconscious always seeks to guard and preserve you from harm of every kind. It will take care of your life and your body if you do not interfere with it by entertaining thoughts of doubt, fear, lack, and limitation.

Millions of people are living lives of mediocrity, lack, and limitation of all kinds because they don't direct their subconscious minds properly. They fail to impregnate their minds with thoughts of harmony, peace, joy, abundance, security, and right action. If you do not direct your subconscious mind according to universal principles and eternal verities, you will then subject it to the thinking of the masses, and this, as you know, is mostly negative.

Begin now to activate your conscious mind spiritually with thoughts of good, and your subconscious will do the rest for you.

Your subconscious does not argue or engage in controversial disputes with your conscious mind's directions, because in the subconscious mind there is only One Power—God, Infinite Intelligence—and there are no divisions or quarrels in this Power. This Power operates by the principle of beauty, not of ugliness; of harmony, not of discord; of love, not of hatred; of joy, not of sadness;

of opulence and abundance, not of deprivation and poverty, of right action, not of wrong action. There can be no antagonism, no quarrels, and no argument where there are only principles of beauty, harmony, love, joy, abundance, and right action.

▓

The fundamental nature of Infinite Intelligence is unity and love. It responds to all your thoughts as if they were moving toward love. This is why your subconscious mind will bring forth whatever thought, plan, or idea you impress upon it, good or bad. It will embrace every thought with love and bring it forth.

▓

Your subconscious mind is in contact with the Universal Subconscious twenty-four hours a day. This contact is never broken. There is always a flow of creative ideas within you, welling up from your Deeper Mind to your conscious mind.

▓

As the residence, the center, the doorway to Infinite Intelligence, your subconscious knows only the answer. It will answer any question, but you must ask without any fear or doubt whatsoever and with assurance that the answer will come in divine order, through divine love.

▓

We may not know everything that is in our subconscious minds, contributing to our lives, but what we're aware of and find harmful, we can change through scientific prayer.

THEY USED THE LAWS OF THE SUBCONSCIOUS

Your subconscious assumptions, convictions, and beliefs dictate and control all your conscious actions by the law of compulsion. This is why your habitual behavior is a function of the subconscious. For example, I was once taken to meet a man in New York City, Al T., who never left his apartment. He would not go out into the street or even down to the lobby of the building. Whenever he planned to leave home, he would imagine all the dire things that might happen to him. He would feel faint and dizzy. This condition is called agoraphobia. The fear originated in Al's early childhood. When he was about five years old, he wandered away from home and was lost in the woods for several hours. His memory of being lost and the anxiety ensuing from it were still lurking in his subconscious mind.

Once, the great operatic tenor Caruso was struck with stage fright. He said his throat was paralyzed due to spasms caused by intense fear, which constricted the muscles of his throat. Perspiration poured copiously down his face. He was ashamed because in a few minutes he had to go out on the stage, yet he was shaking with fear and trepidation. He said, "They will laugh at me. I can't sing." Then he shouted in the presence of those behind the stage, "The Little Me wants to strangle the Big Me within."

It is obvious that Caruso understood the two levels of mind—the conscious and the subconscious.

He then said to the Little Me, "Get out of here; the Big Me wants to sing through me."

By the *Big Me* he meant the limitless power and wisdom of his subconscious mind, and he began to shout, "Get out, get out! The Big Me is going to sing!"

His subconscious mind responded, releasing the vital forces within him. When the call came, he walked out onto the stage and sang gloriously and majestically, enthralling the audience. Your subconscious mind is reactive and responds to the nature of your thoughts. When your conscious mind (the Little Me) is full of fear, worry, foreboding, despair, and a sense of panic, these emotions that you've been planting in your subconscious mind (the Big Me) become who you are. Your subconscious mind then acts on those emotions accordingly and paralyzes you. If you find this happening in your life, you can, like Caruso, speak affirmatively and with a deep sense of authority to the irrational emotions generated in your deeper mind, as follows: "Be still. Be quiet. I am in control. You must obey me. You are subject to my command, you cannot intrude where you do not belong."

As reported in an article in a British newspaper, over a period of about two years a man said, "I would give my right arm to see my daughter cured." His daughter had a crippling form of arthritis, along with a so-called incurable form of skin disease. Medical treatment had failed to alleviate the condition, and the father had an intense longing for his daughter's healing, expressing his desire in the words just quoted.

The newspaper article went on to report that one day, the family was out riding when their car collided with another. The father's right arm was torn off at the shoulder, and immediately the daughter's arthritis and skin condition vanished.

You must make certain to give your subconscious only suggestions that heal, bless, elevate, and inspire you in all your ways. Remember that your subconscious mind cannot take a joke. It takes you at your word.

Techniques for Harnessing the Power of Your Subconscious

Have as clear an idea as possible of what you wish to know or have answered. As you go to sleep at night, say to your subconscious, "Give your attention to this and reveal to me the answer." Say this silently or audibly, whichever appeals to you. When you awaken in the morning, the first thought you have will often be the answer. It may also come in a dream, or flash spontaneously into your conscious mind during the day, when you're preoccupied with something else.

Principles to Remember and Apply

▶ Your subconscious mind does not reason inductively or argue controversially with you. It does not look at two ideas and then make a decision as to which is best. You are to decide that with your conscious mind.

▶ Your subconscious is the storehouse of memory; within your subconscious are recorded all your experiences since childhood. If you can't find or remember something, ask your subconscious and it will reveal the answer to you.

▶ Habit is the function of the subconscious mind. In a very real sense, then, we are creatures of habit. Keep your conscious mind busy with the expectation of the best, and your subconscious will faithfully reproduce your habitual thinking.

▶ Never say, "I am full of fear" or "I am all mixed up." Your subconscious takes these statements literally, and you will remain confused.

▶ Your subconscious magnifies everything you deposit in it. Deposit love, faith, confidence, laughter, and goodwill.

> You live in two worlds: the subjective world of your thoughts, feelings, imagery, beliefs, and opinions; and the objective world from which impressions are conveyed to you through your five senses. The inner controls the outer.

> A changed attitude changes everything. If you have impressed your subconscious with the idea of lack, limitation, and failure, you can immediately reverse the pattern by busying your mind with thoughts of success, prosperity, peace, harmony, and right action.

> The best time to tap the subconscious is prior to sleep, when you are relaxed, at peace, and ready for quietude.

> It is the world within—namely, your thoughts, feelings, and imagery—that makes your world without.

> Your subconscious mind is the source, the residence within you, of Infinite Intelligence and Boundless Wisdom. Trust your subconscious completely. Know that its tendency is always lifeward.

> When you trust the power of your subconscious mind, you always get a response. Keep on seeking and your subconscious mind will respond.

> When you turn over a request to your subconscious, you must do so with confidence and faith that the answer will come.

> When your conscious mind is quiet and receptive, the answer wells up from the Deeper Mind.

> Your subconscious has the answer to all problems. Infinite Intelligence within you knows the answer, and its nature is to respond to your thought. Look within for the answer to your heart's desire.

❭ To live a full and happy life, you must live according to the principles of Cosmic Wisdom. Recognize the One Power, and then your mind will move as a unity.

❭ Learn to use the laws of your mind, and you can attract to yourself wealth, love, happiness, and a life of abundance.

❭ You decree your own security, peace, joy, and health through the laws of your mind.

❭ Your subconscious mind is the source of your ideals, aspirations, and altruistic urges.

2 The Dynamic Power of Your Thoughts and Affirmations

When the words of your mouth and the feeling in your heart agree, nothing will be impossible for you, and you shall reach great heights.

▨

*T*hought is the most powerful force in the universe. It directs the operation of your life, as your subconscious mind does its work according to the orders given it by your conscious mind: your thoughts. This truth is affirmed again and again in the Bible, which says: *As thou hast believed, so be it done unto thee.* (Matthew 8:13)

▨

Thought rules the world. All transactions take place first in the mind.

Everything that *is* must first live in thought-life; nothing can be molded, fashioned, or shaped until it has been thought out. You must first establish the mental equivalent of everything you want in your life.

Your thought has power; it is creative. The tendency of every thought is to manifest itself, and it does so, except as it is neutralized by a more powerful thought of greater intensity.

Every thought is a form of prayer, for the simple reason that every thought is creative, and its tendency is toward action and manifestation.

Thoughts are things. In other words, the mental and the physical interact. An admittedly rather simple way of looking at this interaction between the mental and the physical is to realize that your conscious mind grasps an idea that induces a corresponding vibration in your voluntary system of nerves. This in turn causes a similar current to be generated in your involuntary system of nerves, thus handing the idea over to your subconscious mind, which is the creative medium. This is how your thoughts become things.

Your thought causes the Infinite Power to respond; you are dealing with a reciprocal action-and-reaction: as you sow you reap, and as you call, you receive an answer.

You are thinking in the true sense of the word when you are thinking from the standpoint of universal principles and eternal verities, which never change and are the same yesterday, today, and forever.

If there is any fear, worry, or anxiety in your thoughts, you are not really *thinking*. There is no fear or negation of any kind in *true* thinking. Fear thoughts result when you make external things causative, which is the big lie. Externals are effects. The cause is your thoughts and feelings.

True thinking is thinking from the standpoint of the Truths that never change. It is thinking from the standpoint that in Life, there is a principle of harmony, but none of discord; there is a principle of truth, but none of error; there is a principle of life, but none of death; there is a principle of love, but none of hatred; there is a principle of joy, but none of sadness; there is a principle of opulence, but none of poverty; there is a principle of health, but none of disease; there is a principle of beauty, but none of ugliness; there is a principle of right action, but none of wrong action; there is a principle of light, but none of darkness.

You can think thoughts of fear, worry, resentment, or hate, but in so doing, you would not be thinking in Truth. You would be violating the principles of wholeness, harmony, and love, and you would inevitably reap the consequences.

Respect your thoughts. Think from the standpoint that Truths never change.

Remember: Your thoughts and feelings create your character, and character is destiny.

※

The Bible says *Your thought is your word. Are you words sweet to the ear?* (Proverbs 25:11) and *Pleasant words are as an honeycomb, sweet to the soul, and health to the bones* (Proverbs 16:24) If you say, "I can't get ahead. It is impossible. I'm too old now," "What chance have I to be rich?" "I have no money, I can't afford this," or "I've tried, it's no use," your words are not *as an honeycomb*, they do not lift you up or inspire you. Worse, what you decree in words will actually come to pass.

The words you speak must support your aspirations. Your speech must sustain and strengthen you. Decree now, and say it meaningfully. "From this moment forward, the words I use will heal, bless, prosper, inspire, and so strengthen me."

---

*D*eath and life are in the power of the tongue
(Proverbs 18:21)

Your words are literally so powerful, it is important to say the right thing at the right time.

It is wrong to say, "I am poor", "I am weak", "I am tired", "I am broke." This is not what you *are*, it is the condition you are *bringing on yourself* by your negative "I Am" statements, which become lodged in your subconscious mind as affirmations and which then come forth as experiences and events in your life. It is a mental law that whatever you attach to "I Am," you will manifest and express. Never refer to or describe yourself, therefore, with words of lack, limitation, discord, or bad times. *For by thy words thou shalt be justified and by thy words thou shalt be condemned* (Matthew 12: 37)

Never use the word *can't* under any circumstances. Don't say "I can't make ends meet," "I can't pay the rent," or "I can't afford a new car," as your subconscious mind listens to you literally and will block the flow of your good. Thoughts repeated regularly sink into the subconscious mind and become habitual, as your subconscious treats your self-talk as affirmations.

※

You must never subsequently deny what you affirm, this will neutralize your good. Your affirmations must be embodied in your experience.

※

Be sure that your inner speech agrees with your arm or desire in life. It is your inner speech (your inner conversations, your silent thoughts; affirmations) that will be made manifest.

It is the beginning and cause of the outer experiences in your life.

Ask yourself this question, therefore. "Does my inner speech agree with my aim?" If you answer, "Oh, yes. My inner talking is the same as I would talk aloud were my aims in the fulfilled," you will enter into the joy of the answered prayer.

※

Your words have power to cleanse your mind of wrong ideas and to instill right ideas in their place.

※

Remember—the power of words is one of the greatest that God has bestowed on you. Realize that you can use your words to bless or to curse, to heal or to make sick, to produce riches or poverty, for your betterment or for your detriment. Cease using the power of your words against yourself. Always bless, and then you will gather orchids in life, instead of thistles.

※

If you fix your attention on poverty, lack, loneliness, squalor, meanness, and the difficulties and problems of the world, your mind takes the form of all these things—based on the law that that to which you give attention, you also experience.

※

There is a vast difference between spiritual (Cosmic) thinking and average (mass) thinking. In average thinking, you are not in control of your thought life, and you are not giving correct commands to your subconscious.

Unfortunately, most of us live lives that are the expression of mass thinking: the thoughts and beliefs of others.

Keep your thoughts within Cosmic Consciousness, or you will automatically be a victim of the mass mind. It will do all your thinking for you, resulting in negation and troubles of all kinds for you personally.

※

A man once asked me, "How do I know when I am truly thinking in harmony with Infinite Intelligence?"

This is a good question. The answer is that you are thinking in accord with Infinite Intelligence when you are activating your mind from the standpoint of eternal verities and the Cosmic truths of God, which are the same yesterday, today, and forever. You are *not* thinking, in the true sense of the term, when you are reacting to the headlines in the newspapers, to radio propaganda, or from the standpoint of tradition, dogma, creeds, or environmental conditions or circumstances.

You are truly thinking spiritually when there is no fear or worry in your thought.

※

You can't take credit for your successes and then refuse to assume responsibility for your failures. This is unreasonable and unscientific.

Remember, as you thinketh, so are you—both good and bad.

※

If you are planning something in the future, you are planning it now. Similarly, if you are fearful of something in the future, you are fearing it now. To think of a happy and joyful episode in the past, is a present joy. If you are thinking of the past, you are thinking of it now; if you are thinking of the future, you are thinking of it now.

The past and the future are two thieves. If you are indulging in remorse and self-criticism over past mistakes and hurts, the mental agony you experience is the pain of your present thought.

If you are thinking anxiously about the future, you are robbing and stealing from yourself joy, health, and happiness. Count your blessings now and get rid of the two thieves. Beware of the two thieves. If you are indulging in remorse over past mistakes or are worrying about the future, be aware that the past and future are two thieves that are robbing you of vitality, discernment, and peace of mind.

The only thing you have to change is your present thought.

Your thoughts, beliefs, plans, and purposes and their manifestations are complete in mind, just the same as the idea and manifestations complete of a new building in the mind of the architect. Your thought, idea, plan, or purpose is as real on its own plane as your hand or your heart.

What you experience in the objective world has nothing to do with the way you decide to think about it. You can decide to think in whatever manner you choose about anything.

Your thought carries its own reward. Choose good, and by the immutable law of your subconscious mind, good follows.

Thoughts are things: What you imagine, you become, and what you feel, you attract.

If you do not do your own thinking, the newspapers, the neighbors, and the mass mind will do your thinking for you.

Take charge of your own mind and do not permit others to govern it for you. *Choose you this day whom ye will serve* (Joshua 24: 15).

⬛

Cause is within, in your own thought and feeling. If you are mentally fighting conditions, circumstances, and environmental problems, you are actually making an effect a cause and you are magnifying your troubles and problems, creating your own anxiety.

⬛

You go where your vision is.

Your vision is not just what you are *looking at*, it is what you are giving attention to—that object, idea, or feeling upon which you are presently focused. Whatever you give complete attention to, your subconscious will bring you to. Attention is the key to life.

⬛

Cause and effect, action and reaction, are as absolute and undeviating in the conscious and unconscious realm of thought as in the world of visible and material things. This is why your joy and suffering are the reflections of your habitual thinking.

⬛

Thought becomes a thing in the same way that a seed becomes a plant: by continual nourishment.

⬛

Replacing a false thought with a new thought may at first be just the uttering of an intellectual statement in which emotion and feeling have no part. But with a sincere desire to believe in it, there will come a moment when the last resistance lets go. The repetition of truth by the conscious mind, over and over again, eventually dissolves its opposite and false belief in your subconscious mind.

You do not get what you want in life, you get what you contemplate.

Your current life and your future are your present thoughts made manifest. Your future is in your mind now.

The law is that you become what you contemplate and incorporate into your subconscious. Contemplate love, peace, harmony, joy, beauty, wisdom, power, and guidance, and you will begin to express these qualities.

Your dominant thought underlies all your other thoughts and colors them in the same way a small amount of indigo dye colors the entire contents of a five-gallon jug of water.

William James, the father of American psychology, said, "The greatest discovery of my generation is that human beings can alter their lives by altering their attitudes of mind."

You live in a "thought world." You can experience nothing outside your own mentality.

Thought is the only intangible and invisible power of which you are truly aware and in control. That is how important thought is.

A thought's propensity is to be made manifest, unless the idea is inhibited and neutralized by a counter idea.

Your subconscious mind moves as it is acted upon by your thought.

You live in your mind, and it is there that you become rich or poor, a beggar or a thief.

Your business is with your conscious mind and not your subconscious mind. Your conscious mind is the all-important "guardian at the gate." Its chief function is to protect your subconscious mind from false impressions. Keep your conscious mind busy with the expectation of the best, and make sure the thoughts you habitually think are based on whatsoever things are lovely, true, just, and good.

Select thoughts that bless, heal, inspire, and fill your soul with joy.

Your external actions reveal your inner thought patterns. It is important, therefore, to enthrone in your mind thoughts of peace, harmony, right action, love, and goodwill.

When you begin to control your thought processes, you can mobilize the powers of your subconscious to obtain the solution to any problem or difficulty, as you will actually be consciously cooperating with the Infinite Power and Omnipotent Law that governs all things.

Everything that you find in your world has been created by you in the inner world of your mind, consciously or unconsciously. As Marcus Aurelius, the great Roman emperor and philosopher, said, "Our life is what our thoughts make it."

In order to change your external circumstances, you must work on that principle that is truly causative in your life: thought. Most people try to change their circumstances by working on those circumstances. To remove discord, confusion, lack, and limitation, you must change the cause, and the cause is the way you are using your conscious mind. Change your thoughts, and you won't have to *wish* that your circumstances were different; *you* will change your circumstances.

※

When you reflect on thought and what it truly is, you are releasing the creative power of God, or infinite intelligence, into action.

Your knowledge of the laws of mind counts for little toward your true happiness unless you apply the truths of God to your daily life.

※

Your word is a thought expressed.

※

The creator is greater than his or her creation; the artist is greater than his or her art; the thinker is greater than his or her thoughts. Thus, you can change your thoughts.

※

The five-sense mind, the conscious mind, is the mind that thinks from the standpoint of circumstance, conditions, and traditions. Do not make the external world a cause; it is an effect. Refuse definitely, positively, and absolutely to give power to externals, such as the winds, waves, weather, sun, snow, stars, or any created thing. The scientific thinker never makes an effect a cause; he or she is no longer hypnotized by the world and its beliefs. He or she knows that your mental beliefs are the only cause. Whatever you think, feel, believe, and accept as true in your mind is the only *cause* in your world . . . *it is done unto you as you believe.*

Remember: You are the only thinker in your universe.

Have you questioned the validity and truth of the various ideas and suggestions propounded to you and thought by you during the day?

All your experiences, conditions, and acts are the reactions of your subconscious mind to your thoughts.

If you were building a new home for yourself and your family you would understandably be intensely interested in the blueprint for your home; you would see to it that the builders conformed to the blueprint. You would watch the material and select only the best. What about your mental home and your mental blueprint for it?

All your experiences and everything that enters into your life depend upon the nature of the mental building blocks that you use in the construction of the life you live—what will be, in truth, your personal home. If your blueprint is full of mental patterns of fear, worry, anxiety, or lack, then the mental material you are using in your mind will result in more toil, care, tension, anxiety, and limitation of all kinds.

You are building your mental home all the time. The thoughts you think, the ideas you harbor, the beliefs you accept, and the scenes you rehearse in the hidden studio of your mind are the building materials of your mental home. This stately mansion, the construction of which you are perpetually engaged in hour by hour, moment by moment, is your personality, your destiny, your whole life story on this earth.

THEY USED THE POWER OF THOUGHT TO CHANGE THEIR DESTINIES

A young physicist visited me once and explained that even by modern scientific theories, thoughts could be shown to be things. He pointed out that Einstein and all our modern physicists realize that energy (Spirit) and matter are interconvertible and interchangeable; that as the Hindu Vedas taught generations ago, matter is the lowest degree of Spirit and Spirit is the highest degree of matter. In other words, they are one and the same thing: Matter is Spirit, or energy, reduced to the point of visibility. Thoughts, then, are incipient matter.

The young physicist then demonstrated the evidence of this. He said to me, "When I came to America, all I had was ten dollars, but I didn't get panicky, as I knew the invisible would become visible. I declared in my hotel room, 'Divine Spirit is my instant and everlasting supply. It takes the form of food, clothing, money, friends, and everything I need right here and right now. I decree this and I know the manifestation takes place now, for God is the Eternal Now!' "

His good came to him through a total stranger, whom he met in the hotel elevator. As they conducted a vigorous conversation in French, though both spoke excellent English, the stranger arranged for him to get a position with an electronics research organization, where he eventually became a partner.

The young man who showed up in my office was, frankly, a mess. His name was Bernhart O., and he began by saying, "I got fired yesterday. That makes five jobs in five months. Do you think that's a record?" He went on to tell me he suffered from insomnia, alcoholism, and depression. He seemed almost proud of this recital of problems.

"Why do you think you are fired so often?" I asked.

"They don't like me," he replied. "My bosses, the other people . . . nobody likes me. Maybe it's my face, or something chemical."

"Are you a good worker?" I probed. "Do you show up every day on time and put a real effort into your job?"

He looked away. "It's not my fault," he mumbled. "Sometimes I just don't feel up to going. If I've been up all night, not able to sleep."

"Or suffering from a terrible hangover?" I suggested.

"Yeah, that, too," he said. "Anyway, what's the use? They're not going to like me, whatever I do, and sooner or later I'll get fired."

I explained to Bernhart that his dominant thoughts of pessimism and helplessness were coloring everything, and that correspondingly, of course, his bosses didn't care for him and didn't keep him. Why should they? He gave them nothing and could expect nothing in return.

At my suggestion, Bernhart took a course in business fundamentals and another course in public speaking. He began to pray for guidance and prosperity, claiming regularly that God was guiding him in all his ways and that he was prospered beyond his fondest dreams.

Gradually Bernhart's underlying thoughts changed. He acquired confidence; he began to express health, harmony, happiness, and true living. In his next job, he was kept on after a probation period and soon was promoted to greater responsibilities.

Bernhart learned that practically all teaching—whether institutional, religious, or secular—has for its real purpose the inducement of a changed mental attitude toward life, people, and events. The first step in his onward march was correcting his thought-life.

The credit manager of an engineering firm had many delinquent accounts, totaling nearly $30,000. He made a list of past-due accounts and every morning before he started to work he mentioned each name and spoke the words as follows. "John Doe is prospered and blessed, and his good is multiplied. He pays all his obligations promptly and he is honest, sincere, and just. I give thanks now for his check. He is blessed, we are blessed. I give thanks that it is so."

This statement, or command to the credit manager's deeper mind reached each one of his customers who had been very lax, and all paid within one month! His words of faith and trust were accepted by his subconscious mind and were telepathically received by those men who had been in arrears and who had previously failed to answer his frequent requests for payment.

Change your thoughts, realize that thoughts and not conditions are the cause, and you can change your destiny.

A Technique for Using the Power of Your Thoughts

The late Dr. Dan Custer, who lectured on the Science of the Mind for many years in San Francisco, practiced what he termed the "therapy of words." For example, if he felt tense, he would repeat silently the word *Peace* over and over again. When fearful or anxious about something, he would silently affirm, "Indomitability." And when an acute problem presented itself, he would say, "Victory" over and over again.

Dr. Custer said that the practice of repeating these words worked magic throughout his life. As he invoked these words, he was actually stirring up the latent powers of his subconscious mind, and these powers became active and potent factors in his life.

Repeating an affirmation of your good, knowing what you are saying and why you are saying it, *and regardless of all the evidence to the contrary*, leads to that state of consciousness where your subconscious accepts that which you state as true. Keep on affirming the truths of life until you get the subconscious reaction which satisfies.

Take certain words whose implications appeal to you and verbally decree them over and over for about ten or more minutes twice daily—for example, "Health. Wealth. Happiness. Love." If you work in close proximity to others and feel you cannot always affirm out loud, write down what it is that you are wishing to bring to pass and mentally go over your statements from time to time, thereby gradually conveying the ideas to your subconscious mind.

You are the sum total of your own thoughts. Today you are what your thoughts have made you. The results of past events—good or bad—are but the representatives of your present thinking.

Just as the way to get rid of darkness is with light and the way to overcome cold is with heat, the way to overcome a negative thought is with a good thought. Affirm the good, and the bad will vanish; affirm the true, and the false will vanish.

Principles to Remember and Apply

▶ Thoughts repeatedly sent to your subconscious are accepted as true and brought into reality. If you consciously dwell on obstacles, delays, and difficulties, your subconscious mind responds accordingly, and you are blocking your own good. *How* do you *think*?

▶ True thinking is when your thoughts are God-like, when you are thinking from the standpoint of universal principles and eternal truths. You are not really thinking when there is any fear, doubt, or worry in your thinking.

▶ To affirm is to state that it is so, and as you maintain this attitude of mind as true, regardless of all evidence to the contrary, you will receive an answer to your prayer.

▶ Your conscious mind is the "guardian at the gate." Its chief function is to protect your subconscious mind from false impressions.

▶ When your attention wanders, bring it back to the contemplation of your good or your goal. This is called disciplining the mind.

▶ Your mental attitude (thought and feeling) is *cause*, and your experience is *effect*. This can also be stated in terms of action and reaction: The action is your thought, and the reaction is the response of your subconscious mind.

▶ The cause of all the trouble in your life is due to the kind of company you are keeping in your mind. Take inventory now.

▶ Use words that appeal to you, that fascinate and enthrall you, and repeat them frequently. It is the frequent habitation of the mind with these thoughts that produces miracles in your life.

❱ There are infinite riches within your subconscious mind. Think of harmony, peace, joy, love, guidance, right action, and success. Your subconscious will compel you to express the abundant life right here and right now, because thoughts are things.

❱ You go where your vision (thinking) is. Whatever you give attention to, your subconscious will magnify and multiply in your experience. Understand at all times that your subconscious listens to and answers your word, which it treats as your conviction.

❱ What you affirm, you must not mentally deny a few moments later. This will neutralize the good you have affirmed. When a thought comes to you, such as "I can't afford a new car," affirm immediately, "Wealth is mine now," again and again. After a while the positive idea will be impressed in your subconscious mind.

❱ Your thought is energy. If your thoughts are God's thoughts, God's power is with your thoughts of good.

❱ Change your thought now, and you change everything, because your thoughts can create. It doesn't matter how often you may have used your mind in a negative and destructive manner. The minute you begin to use it in the right way, right results follow. This knowledge will deliver you from countless fears and worries.

❱ Realize that whatever you attach to "I Am" you will create in your life. Have a little phrase that can be easily engraved on your memory, such as "I am happy, joyous, free," etc. Repeat it over and over again knowingly and feelingly, and as you sow in your subconscious, so also will you reap.

‣ Infinite Intelligence in your subconscious can only do *for* you what it can do *through* you. Ultimately, therefore, it is your thoughts and feelings that control your destiny.

‣ Your inner speech must conform to your aim or desire in life. Be certain that your inner talking is the same as it would be if your prayers were answered now.

3 The Amazing Power of Belief and Faith

Whatever you mentally accept and feel to be true,
will come to pass.

※

You are, in reality, invisible. The real you cannot be seen by others. Everything you are, appear to be, and have become is a manifestation of your faith—and your faith is in the unseen.

※

Belief is one thing and thought is another. If you *think* of a successful achievement, but *believe* you are going to fail, it is your belief of failure that will be made manifest.

Your faith, then, is that which you become, because you manifest and objectify in your world what you really believe about yourself.

※

The law of life is belief, and belief could be summed up briefly as a thought in your mind. The importance of this law cannot be overestimated, as it is done unto you as you believe.

What, *right now*, do you believe about yourself, about life, about the universe?

The answer is what your life is for you in this very moment, because we demonstrate our faith. For better or for worse, we are always demonstrating and manifesting that in which we *believe*.

When I speak of faith—*and even as it is spoken of in the Bible*—I am not referring to creeds, dogmas, traditions, rituals, ceremonies, institutions, formulas, religious persuasion, or belief in a particular person, object, or thing. Look upon faith as an attitude of mind, an inner certitude—a certain way of thinking whereby you know that any idea that you emotionalize and feel to be true, *is* true and will be shown to *be* true.

What is faith?

Saint Paul said, *Faith is the substance of things hoped for; the evidence of things not seen.* (Hebrews 11:1)

Saint Augustine said, "For what is faith unless it is to believe what you do not see?"

Faith is perceiving the *reality* of an idea, thought, or image in your mind. You have faith when you know that the idea of a book, play, composition, or invention in your mind is as real as your hand or heart. This is *the substance of things hoped for; the evidence of things not seen.* Others are not able to see the new invention in your mind, but as you accept it and give it attention, the law of growth will take place. It is like the seed in the ground; you cannot see it, but as you nurture and nourish it, it grows.

Faith, then, is accepting as true what your reason and senses deny. It is shutting out the rational, analytical, conscious mind and embracing an attitude of complete reliance on the inner power of your subconscious mind.

Faith is in the invisible.

A chemist has faith in the laws of chemistry, having learned the principles of chemistry; a farmer has faith in the laws of agriculture, having learned the principles of agriculture; and an engineer has faith in the laws of mathematics, having learned the principles of mathematics. To live the life you truly desire, you must have faith in the laws of your mind, having first learned the principles of your conscious and subconscious mind.

Faith is a way of thinking, a confidence in the creative laws of your mind.

The subconscious mind will bring to pass any picture held in the mind and backed by faith.

You increase your faith when you realize that your desire is real, even though invisible. To know with certainty that your idea is real, that it is already a fact in your mind, will give you faith and enable you to rise above doubt to a place of conviction deep in your heart.

Faith is a way of thinking. It is a constructive mental attitude or a feeling of confidence that what you desire will come to pass.

※

Actually, when you stop to look around you and think about it, it is obvious that everything accomplished in this world is done so by faith. You do *everything* by faith. You bake a cake and you drive your car by the faith in your ability to do so.

※

Everyone has faith in something. Some people have faith in failure, sickness, accidents, and misfortune. When you hear exhortations to have faith, you must remember that you already have faith. The question is, how are you using it constructively or negatively?

※

You have faith when you know—that is, accept as true—that thoughts are things; that what you feel, you attract; and that what you imagine, you become.

※

There is a law of cause and effect operating at all times, such that nothing happens to you without your mental consent and participation. You do not have to *think* of an accident to have it befall you. If at some level you are holding the belief that you *might* have an accident, then sooner or later it will happen. The truth is that we demonstrate what we *really believe*.

More than a century ago, Dr. Phineas Parkhurst Quimby of Maine set this point forth as a simple and wonderful psychological truth. He said that if you believe something, it will become manifest, whether you are consciously thinking of it or not.

※

It is done unto you as you believe. In other words, everything you do happens automatically according to your belief.

※

The law of your mind is the law of belief. This does not mean that you should therefore give your wholehearted belief to external circumstances, events, or conditions as causes. It means *to believe in the way your mind works: to understand that your mind works by belief—that is, in accordance with what you believe—so that you have profound belief in the very power of belief.*

To truly understand belief, therefore, is to understand the principle of your mind—that is, the way your mind works. To say that the law of your mind is the law of belief, then, is to say that your mind works by and through your beliefs. Know this, and you will have acquired a profound wisdom and the key to achieving all of your goals.

※

The belief of your mind is the thought in your mind, just that and nothing else. As you understand the power of belief, you understand the importance of watching your thoughts.

※

To believe is to accept something as true. Many, however, accept as true that which is absolutely false; consequently, they suffer to the extent of their beliefs. You can believe a falsehood. So, for example you believe that Los Angeles is in Arizona. But if you address your letter accordingly, it will not reach its destination.

⸬

The word *believe* is made up of two words, *be alive*. The old English meaning of the word is to "live in the state of being," which means making it real in your life. To believe means to make alive your conceived truths, feel the reality of them in your heart. It is much more than a conscious or theoretical assent; it means that you must *feel* the truth of what you affirm in your heart.

For you to truly express faith in something, your "head knowledge" must become "heart knowledge."

Then you not only believe, you *demonstrate* your belief.

⸬

To accept an idea is to actually believe it.

⸬

Faith is a mental image that in time clothes itself in a body of manifestation.

⸬

Our beliefs are our masters.

⸬

The law of belief operates in all religions of the world and is the reason they all are psychologically true. The Buddhist, the Christian, the Muslim, and the Jew all are able to receive answers to their prayers—but not because of the particular creed, religion, affiliation, ritual, ceremony, formula, liturgy, incantation, sacrifices, or offerings, but solely because of their belief, or mental acceptance and receptivity, about that for which they pray.

As a person thinks, feels, and believes, so it is done unto him or her.

Our lives are the result of the totality of our beliefs. That is why the law of life is the law of belief.

Your subconscious mind works according to the law of belief. All things that have happened to you are based on the thoughts you've impressed on your subconscious mind through belief.

What you believe in decides how you will live.

To believe is to accept something as true; thus, be mindful of what you believe, for as the sixteenth-century Swiss physician and alchemist Paracelsus said: "Whether the object of your faith be true or false, you will get the same results." In other words, you will bring it to pass.

*F*aith without works is dead. (James 2:26)

This means that if there were not results, faith would be meaningless.

Have unwavering faith in there being a Principle of Life that responds to your belief and never fails you. You will then see the *works* (results) of your faith in your mind, body, and affairs. You will see the *works* of your faith appearing in all your undertakings, be they professional or personal.

The fruits (*works*) of faith come in accordance with the nature of your faith. Have faith in there being a Principle of Life that responds to your belief and never fails you, and the fruits of your faith will be health, happiness, peace, love, goodwill, abundance, security, poise, balance, serenity, and tranquillity.

Many people affirm a belief in a system of theology or certain ecclesiastical dogmas, but they have no workable faith at all in their lives and their lives are quite chaotic. Your faith, to be real, must be personally demonstrated in your mind, body, and affairs.

Whatever you think, feel, believe, and accept as true in your mind is the only *cause* in your world. Remember: *It is done unto you as you believe.*

SPIRITUAL, OR TRUE, FAITH

A man once said to me, "I had absolute faith that my thoroughbred would win the race." His horse, it turned out, had dropped dead in the race!

I explained to him that it is impossible to have *absolute faith* in anything but the principles of life and the working of the laws of one's subconscious mind. Principles and laws never change—they are eternal, immutable, and timeless.

It is impossible to have absolute faith in any event, circumstance, or condition in life. The Bible is replete with stories of those who put their faith in externals—for example, Adam and Eve in a snake, the children of Israel in a golden calf, Samson in Delilah—rather than in the Unchanging Truth, and consequently suffered loss.

Your faith should be in God, His Cosmic gifts, and in all things good. With that accomplished, success, prosperity, and happiness will be assured you in ways you know not of.

Faith in its true meaning is the practice of the presence of God within you.

Place your faith in God and all things good, and you will attract to yourself—by an immutable law—the people, conditions, circumstances, and events in the image and likeness of your contemplation.

When you know that the light and love of God are guiding and governing you in all your ways, you know that you cannot make errors in judgment or unwise decisions, or waste your time and efforts on useless endeavors.

Faith is a way of thinking whereby you think from the standpoint of principles and eternal truths. Faith can be looked upon as a constructive mental attitude or as a feeling of confidence and assurance that what you are praying for will come to pass.

Two excellent examples of the power of true faith are stated in the Bible:

And what shall I more say? For the time would fail me to tell of Gedeon, and of Barak, and of Samson, and of Jephthae; of David also, and Samuel, and of the prophets: Who through faith subdued kingdoms, wrought righteousness, obtained promises, stopped the mouths of lions, quenched the violence of fire, escaped the edge of the sword, out of weakness were made strong, waxed valiant in fight, turned to flight the armies of aliens. (Hebrews 11:32–34)

For verily I say unto you, That whosoever shall say unto this mountain, Be thou removed, and be thou cast into the sea; and shall not doubt in his heart, but shall believe that those things which he saith shall come to pass; he shall have whatsoever he saith. (Mark 11:23)

It is the belief you hold in your mind that determines the difference between success and failure, health and sickness, happiness and unhappiness, joy and sadness, wealth and poverty. To lead a life of health, happiness, right action, and prosperity, your faith must be only in a God of love, the Infinite Intelligence and Boundless Wisdom, which is the Ever-Living One, the All-Knowing One, and the All-Powerful One.

Have faith in the Eternal Principle of Life within you, which created you and is never-changing.

Theologies, philosophies, governmental operations, and fiscal values wax and wane, come and go. Governments topple, wars and strife cause money to lose its value. Sometimes floods, hurricanes, and other cataclysms of nature sweep away cities, towns, and homes. Everything in this world passes away and is subject to change, except the Principle of Life—God—which remains the same yesterday, today, and forever.

Belief and expectancy stir up the dormant powers in the depths of your subconscious mind, which were always there, waiting to be recognized and utilized.

*W*herefore, I put thee in remembrance, that thou stir up the gift of God, which is in thee. (II Timothy 1:6)

Most people are asleep to the God Power and the God Wisdom locked in their unconscious depths, so they daily do battle with the events and conditions in the world.

Persons of faith awaken and stir up the gift of God within them. They know that their ideals or desires are real in the Inner Kingdom, and that their faith or feeling will cause the invisible

Presence to take on substance as a condition, event, or experience. This is why the person of faith walks upon the waters of doubt and fear and moves in confidence and understanding to the promised land—his or her cherished goal.

Faith is a way of thinking. It is a constructive mental attitude or a feeling of confidence that what you are praying for or desire will come to pass because of Infinite Intelligence operating within you. To truly have faith, you must have unwavering conviction in there being a Principle of Life that responds to your thought and never fails you.

For verily I say unto you, If ye have faith as a grain of mustard seed . . . nothing shall be impossible unto you. (Matthew 17:20)

If you claim that you do not believe in universal principles and the truths of God, but in some subsequent circumstance in your life you find yourself affirming that what is true of God is true of you, then the mere fact that you began, even ever so slightly, to affirm this truth is the *faith as a grain of mustard seed*—and it will expand and grow as you continue to reiterate and announce this truth to your mind. And you will discover that belief works wonders, and even miracles, in your life.

The noblest, grandest, and highest faith is based on eternal principles that never change. Have faith in the creative law of your own mind, in all things good, and in a joyous expectancy of the best. Have the firm belief inscribed in your heart in the invisible Intelligence within you, which created you and is all-powerful, and which will lead you out of any difficulty and show you the way. This faith will enable you to walk over the waters of fear, doubt, worry, and imaginary dangers of all kinds.

TRUE FAITH VERSUS BLIND FAITH

True faith consists in knowing that the Infinite Presence that created you from a cell knows all, and certainly knows how to heal you of any ailment—be it of the body, the heart, or the pocketbook.

What is popularly termed faith healing is not the faith mentioned in the Bible, which is knowledge of the interaction of the conscious and subconscious mind. A faith healer may be any person who heals without any real scientific understanding of the powers and forces involved. Faith healers claim to have a special gift of healing, but it is the sick person's blind belief in either the healer or his or her powers that is actually producing the results.

When you consciously tune in to the healing power of your subconscious, knowing and believing that it will respond to you and that you will get results, you are exercising true faith. True faith, in other words, is the combined, cooperative, and reciprocal use of your conscious and subconscious mind, scientifically directed for a specific purpose.

In 1776 the Swiss physician Franz Anton Mesmer claimed many cures when he stroked diseased bodies with artificial magnets. Later on he threw away his magnets and evolved the theory of animal magnetism. This he held to be a fluid that pervades the universe, but was most active in the human organism.

He claimed that this magnetic fluid, which was going forth from him to his patients, healed them. People flocked to him, and many wonderful cures were effected. Mesmer moved to Paris, and while he was there the government appointed a commission composed of physicians and members of the Academy of Science, of which Benjamin Franklin was a member, to investigate his cures. The report admitted the leading facts claimed by Mesmer, but held that there was no evidence to prove the correctness of his magnetic fluid theory, and said the effects were due to the imagination of the patients. Soon after this, Mesmer was driven into exile.

Perhaps the most revealing clue as to the operation of blind faith is in the fact that our word *mesmerize*—meaning to hypnotize—is derived from Mesmer's name. To hypnotize is to get another to act on the basis of the hypnotizer's suggestion. It is getting a person to act on the basis of the hypnotizer's appeal to act. That, in a nutshell, is how blind faith works.

THE POWER OF FAITH WORKED FOR THEM

While lecturing in San Francisco, I met Arthur R., the general manager of a large corporation. He confided to me that he had lost confidence in himself. He was very unhappy and dejected over the way his career was going.

"I report to two people," he explained, "the executive vice president and the CEO. Both of them keep opposing me. Whatever I suggest, they're against it automatically. Between them, they are driving the firm into the ground. Before long my stock options will be worthless. I'll have wasted five years of my life. And the worst part is, I have absolutely no faith in my ability to do anything about it."

"Unless you are willing to put your confidence in the invisible powers within you," I told him, "whatever you do is going to go badly."

"Invisible powers!" he scoffed. "I'm sorry. I don't mean to belittle your beliefs. I'm sure you're very sincere. But as for me, I believe in what I can see, hear, touch, taste, or smell. I don't have room in my system for mystical ideas."

I smiled and responded, "I understand. Many people feel the same way. But where do they feel that way? Can you pin down the location of their skepticism?"

"Why, it's in their minds, I suppose," he replied. "You're going to ask me where my mind is. All right. I have to admit, I don't know exactly."

"But you know you have one," I said.

"Unless I've lost it," he joked.

"Do you have children?" I asked. He nodded. "Do you love them? Can you see that love? Or only its effects in the world? It is the same with the Infinite Intelligence that is within you and every person. We cannot see it, we cannot locate it, but we can see its effects in the world."

As we continued to talk, Arthur came to realize that in order to advance in business and to have peace of mind and success, he had to anchor himself to a wisdom and a power that transcended his intellect. He had to get in touch with that which is substantial and eternal. He made a deliberate decision to unite mentally and emotionally with the inner power lodged in his subconscious mind.

I later received a letter from Arthur. At the end of two weeks, the CEO and the vice president met with him privately. Each shook hands with him and said that the organization could not get along without his creative energies.

His faith was restored.

I once explained to a woman that the only thing you cannot have in life is something for nothing. She had been praying for a healing of a skin condition for ten years with no results. She had applied various astringent lotions and other topical medication, without any appreciable relief.

But she had never paid the price for healing: faith—faith in the Infinite Healing Presence, for "according to your faith is it done unto you." Faith is attention, devotion, and loyalty to the One Creative Power, the Living Spirit Almighty within, which created all things. The price this woman had to pay was recognition of the power of God, acceptance of His Healing Presence, and conviction that the healing is taking place now.

She had been giving power to externals, saying, "My skin is sensitive to the sun"; "I am allergic to the cold weather, also"; "I believe this eczema all over my arm is a hereditary condition"; "It's my genes and chromosomes that are at fault."

Her mind was divided, which she acknowledged with these words: "I could have anything I want, if I would only believe I had it in my mind." She had never paid the price for healing, which was to give her attention to God and His laws, to trust Him and believe in Him and that He would bring her healing to pass.

You must give before you can get. You must put the seed in

the ground to get a harvest. Likewise, you must first impress your subconscious mind with the belief of what it is you desire. You must let the Universal Energy flow through your ideals, hopes, and aspirations, vitalizing and energizing them. Then you will feel the joy of answered prayer.

A Technique for Using the Power of Belief

If you believe it, it will come to pass. Here is an example of how this truth can work in your life.

If you want to take a trip and do not have a penny in your pocket, believe that you will have the answer to your desire and then take some action that will indicate that you have faith that your prayer is already answered in your deeper mind. For example, adopt the mental attitude of being already in the country or on the plane; have your passport and bags ready and all other requirements needed for overseas travel.

Principles to Remember and Apply

▶ Know that what you believe in your heart (subconscious mind) becomes your life.

▶ Faith is accepting as true that which your reason and senses deny. Believe the riches of the infinite power within your conscious and you will experience them.

▶ Faith is a mental attitude that commands and gets results.

▶ To believe something is to accept it as true. This simple truth is of great consequence, because whatever you mentally accept and feel to be true will come to pass.

▶ You do not need more faith; you have plenty of faith, but you must use it constructively. Give it purposeful direction. Have faith in health, success, peace, and happiness.

❯ It is not what you profess to believe with your lips that matters. What matters is the belief deep down in your heart that is made manifest.

❯ All things that have happened to you are based on the thoughts you've impressed on your subconscious mind through belief. What you believe in decides how you will live.

❯ True faith consists of the belief that the Infinite Presence that created you knows all the processes and functions of your body, and that when you unite with It believingly, results will follow.

❯ Your faith must be placed in the guidance of God, in the love of God, in the harmony of God, and in Divine law and order. Real faith must be placed in the workings of your conscious and subconscious mind and in the truths of God, which never change.

❯ Believe in the reality of your idea, plan, or invention; believe that the idea you have is real in your mind and that you can have it now; and as you do, it will become manifest. Have faith in the creative laws of your mind, which never fail and never change.

❯ You must have a workable and working faith. It must be demonstrated in your home, in your relationships with people, and in your finances. Faith without demonstration and results is dead.

❯ It is done unto you as you believe.

❯ Mentally act and feel the way you would act and feel were your prayer(s) answered, and you will find that the power of faith will work wonders in your life.

❯ You can't get something for nothing. The price you pay for answered prayer is faith—faith in the Infinite Wisdom, the Infinite Healing within you—for according to your faith is it done unto you.

4 The Miraculous Power of Prayer

Prayer is always the solution.

◼

*H*ere is a typical dialogue about prayer:

"How long should my prayer be?"

"You should pray until you feel satisfied within, or you feel that what you've done is the best you can do for the time being. A short prayer uttered from the heart gets better results than a long prayer. Long sessions of prayer are usually a mistake, as they may indicate you are trying to force things by using mental coercion, which always results in the opposite of what you are praying for."

"What steps should I take after I have the belief that my prayer will be answered?"

"Nothing. You don't aid Infinite Intelligence."

Prayer is the greatest force in all the world! Consider what we are told: *Whatsoever ye shall ask in prayer, believing, ye shall receive.* (Matthew 21:22) We have been told, then—and daily proofs support this—that when we believingly invoke the blessings, protection, and guidance of the Infinite Intelligence, the answer will come.

In other words, no matter what the problem might be, no matter how great the difficulty or how complicated the matter seems to be, prayer can solve it and bring about a happy and joyous solution—if in your praying you conform to the laws of your mind purposefully, sincerely, and righteously.

When you pray, you are not praying to a God "out there;" you are praying to the Healing Presence that is *within and throughout* you. You are focusing your attention on the Healing Presence within, to mobilize its powers to assist you in bringing about some desired change—some healing of body, mind, spirit, relationship, finances, or whatever.

If someone asked me how I pray, I would respond by saying that to me, prayer means the contemplation of the eternal verities or truths of the Infinite from the highest possible standpoint. It's a way of thinking. It is a constructive mental attitude with the constant awareness that whatever you impress on your subconscious mind will come forth on the screen of space.

In other words, prayer is belief.

No matter what you are praying for, if it is God-ward and brings no harm to others, it already is, for all things good and noble subsist in the Infinite within you. The answers exist now and are awaiting your call and recognition. All you have to do is to claim, feel, know, and believe that the answer is yours now, and the solution will come.

You can know if you have succeeded in prayer by the way you feel: If you remain worried or anxious, and are wondering how, when, where, or through what source your answer will come, or you think that "just to be sure," you'd best pray "one more time," this indicates you are not yet trusting the Wisdom of your subconscious. You are meddling. Learn to relinquish authority to your subconscious mind.

Go to sleep believing you have the answer *now*. Do not postulate the answer in the future. Have an abiding faith in the outcome. Be convinced that there is an answer and a perfect solution for you.

If there seems to be an undue delay in getting the answer to your prayer, do not be discouraged. You will not always get an answer to your prayer overnight. Ask that Infinite Intelligence reveal to you what more you need to know. It will. Then simply gently turn the problem over to the subconscious mind every night prior to sleep, as if you had never done it before.

And by all means, cease pestering your subconscious. Mentally devote yourself to the right answer. Quiet your body, tell it to be still and relax, and it will obey you. It is the quiet mind that gets things done. When your conscious mind is quiet and receptive, the wisdom of your subconscious mind rises to the surface mind and you will know that you are receiving the answer to your prayer.

You will know your prayer is answered when you experience an inner sense of peace and certitude, followed by no further desire to pray.

※

Effective prayer consists in your degree of conviction of the spiritual premise that there is an Infinite Intelligence within you that becomes the thing you desire.

※

Prayer constantly brings about the seemingly impossible and heals the so-called incurable.

※

The answer to prayer comes not from your devout investment of power in some external condition, circumstance, event, or person. The answer to prayer is the result of your subconscious mind responding to the mental picture or thought *in your mind*.

※

Many people's prayers aren't answered because consciously or unconsciously they are believing in two powers, or forces, in the world: one that brings sickness, and one that brings health; one that brings success, and one that brings failure; one that brings joy, and one that brings sorrow.

You will never be truly effective in prayer until you awaken to the greatest of all truths, expressed in Deuteronomy 6:4: *Hear, O Israel: The Lord our God is one.*

There is but One Power. Know this in your heart, and you will gain confidence and cease struggling, straining, and believing that you must put great effort into your prayers—thinking that praying is a type of contest between opposing forces.

Here is one of the great truths of the power of prayer: Through prayer, you can change your subconscious mind from reproducing erroneous thought-patterns and habits in your life.

In prayer, you are communing with your subconscious mind. When you offer *new* mental patterns to your subconscious mind through prayer, the latter accepts the new imagery and the past is obliterated and expunged.

*P*ray without ceasing. (I Thessalonians 5:17)

This does not mean that you pray all day long; instead, it means that you ceaselessly think constructively and lovingly, re-membering that your thoughts are your prayers.

Prayer is the law of substitution made manifest. Prayer is sub-stituting for the challenge, the fear, the worry, or the doubt you're facing, an abiding faith in the Law of God, which organizes the universe and all the workings of your body and in which there is no fear, no challenge, no worry, no doubt.

Never once permit your mind to wander after false gods (negative beliefs). If you do, you will rob yourself of your strength and faith, nullifying your prayer.

When you pray, you must sincerely believe that you have the right to your heart's desire.

Prayer is conscious contact with the Infinite Intelligence within you.

In truth, *you* answer your own prayer, whether you are aware of it or not, because whatever you really believe to be true and accept in your conscious mind, *is already real.* In your mind, in other words, it is already a reality. Your subconscious mind simply brings it forth consistently as form, function, experience, and events.

Prayer is an act of spiritual companionship: Your conscious mind is conversing with your Higher Self, the God Presence within you, whereupon your Higher Self responds according to your belief in it.

The very fact that you desire an answer means that the answer is already present in your mental and spiritual world. *Before they call, I will answer; and while they are yet speaking, I will hear.* (Isaiah 65:24)

You must cast out of your mind all doubts, false beliefs, superstitions, and previous notions, realizing that with regard to prayer, *"All things be ready if the mind be so."*

You must order your mind and thoughts to conform to the age-old truth that whatever you are seeking already subsists in Infinite Mind. All you have to do is identify mentally and emotionally with your desire, idea, plan, or purpose, realizing *it is already as real as your hand or heart.*

In order to receive an answer to your prayer, you must first give to your mind. When you pray, you are not supplicating some distant deity. You are activating the Infinite Intelligence resident within you to begin working on behalf of your expressed desires.

The farmer has to deposit seeds in the ground in order to get a harvest. He or she has to give in order to get. Similarly, to receive your prayer's answer, you must first plant in the ground of your subconscious mind the idea of what it is you desire. Then, whatever is impressed will become expressed.

Real prayer is not begging, beseeching, or supplicating. When you understand the laws of your own mind, you realize that it is foolish to think that you have to beg for something already given to you. The wisdom of your subconscious mind already knows the answer to your prayer. It has no problem. Consider for a moment: If Infinite Intelligence (your subconscious mind) had a problem, who would solve it?

Moreover, begging, beseeching, and supplicating would be attempting to change God. When you pray, you should not be trying to change the Infinite Source of All, which is God—for God is the same yesterday, today, and forever. You are praying to bring about a change in you, in your state of mind and being, so that some desired goal can be achieved. Effective prayer is aligning yourself with that which is true of God and which through you becomes a focal point for the expression of life, love, truth, beauty, joy, and abundance in your life. In other words, prayer is the contemplation of the truths of God from the highest standpoint.

When you beg and beseech, you are expressing that you don't have what you want now, and your sense of lack attracts more loss, lack, and limitation.

All you have to do is call on the wisdom of your subjective mind with faith and confidence, knowing that whatever idea you claim and feel to be true will be impressed on your subconscious and will come to pass from the depths of yourself.

The God you are beseeching has already given you everything. You are here to appropriate and meditate on the reality of your idea or desire. Rejoice and give thanks, knowing that as you contemplate the reality of your desire, idea, plan, or purpose, your subconscious will bring it to pass. Be a good receiver. The gifts of God have been given to you from the foundation of time.

The principal reasons for prayer failure are lack of confidence from not fully understanding the law of the subconscious mind, and too much effort.

You must remember that whenever your subconscious mind accepts an idea, it immediately begins to execute it. That is answered prayer, and that is why I have said that our thoughts are our prayers.

Failure to get results from prayer often arises from praying for one thing while simultaneously expressing such thoughts as, "Things are getting worse," "I will never get an answer," "I see no way out," "It is hopeless," "I don't know what to do," "I'm all mixed up."

If expressed with conviction, these thoughts will be accepted by your subconscious mind instead of your prayer, as your subconscious is always controlled by the dominant idea. It will always accept the stronger of two contradictory propositions.

That is why, before you express a prayer, you must arrive at a definite decision that there is a way out from the concern you are praying about. If you keep giving your subconscious mind conflicting information, it is like getting into a taxi and giving half a dozen different directions to the driver in five minutes. He or she would become hopelessly confused and probably would refuse to take you anywhere. Your subconscious will respond identically.

"Knock, and it shall be opened unto you." (Matthew 7:7) This means that when you have come to a clear-cut and definite decision in your conscious mind about what it is you are seeking in your prayer, you will gain a response from your deeper mind, which is full of wisdom and power.

To overcome the failure in prayer caused by giving your subconscious mind conflicting, worrisome, or negative thoughts, *feel* the reality of your answered prayer. Take your mind off the concerns. Remind yourself how you felt after you recovered from a severe illness. Occupy your conscious mind with *the feel of the happy solution to your problem now*—whether it is health, finances, or employment. Remember that *feeling* is the touchstone of all subconscious demonstration.

If you find your intellect trying to get in the way, continue picturing yourself without the problem. Imagine the emotional accompaniment of the freedom state you crave. Persist in maintaining a simple, childlike, miracle-making faith.

When there is no longer any quarrel in either part of your mind, when you turn over your request with faith and confidence, when you come to that clear-cut conclusion in your conscious mind and you imagine the reality of the fulfilled desire and feel the thrill of accomplishment, your mind is made up, and your subconscious will then bring about the realization of your desire.

According to your belief is it done unto you.

<hr />

You do not succeed in prayer by rushing, hurrying, struggling, straining, or using mental coercion of any kind. Trying to force your subconscious to do something is like telling yourself, "I must have this problem solved by Saturday. It's extremely important."

Have you ever had the experience of finding that the name of a certain person or song or film has suddenly deserted you? Your mind becomes appallingly blank, and you are unable to recall anything associated with what you are trying to remember. The more you grit your teeth and summon the powers of the will, the further the answer seems to flee. But then, when you have left the setting where the information was desired and the mental pressure relaxes, the answer you were seeking flows tantalizingly back into your mind. Trying to force yourself to remember was the cause of your failure.

Avoid struggle and strain, since this attitude is indicative of your unbelief. In your subconscious is all the wisdom and power necessary to solve any problem. It is your conscious mind that is prone to look at external conditions and doubt and think that it must continually struggle.

You will always fail to get results by trying to use mental

coercion. Your subconscious mind does not respond to coercion. It responds to your faith—or your conscious mind's acceptance.

Prayer is cooperation with your subconscious. Lightness of touch is important. Remind yourself that Infinite Intelligence is taking care of things in Divine order far better than you can by tenseness of your conscious mind. With the subconscious mind, relaxation is the key.

Do not be concerned with details and means as to how your prayer will be answered. Turn your request over quietly, with faith and confidence, to your subconscious mind, knowing in your heart that the answer will come—knowing that like the seed you deposit in the ground, which grows after its kind, so will there be an answer to your request according to your desire.

Only Infinite Intelligence within your subconscious knows the answer. Imagine the end as finished state. The law of your mind will do the rest.

You can pray for another. When doing so, you are claiming that what is true of God in you is true also of the person for whom you pray. You aren't trying to send healing thoughts to the other person regarding his or her problem (for example, "I now will that Sally's problem is resolved"). You are instead affirming, identifying with, and thereby activating the Divine Presence in the other (for example, "I know that Infinite Intelligence is in Sally and can resolve her problem"). In this way, you are affirming resurrecting the qualities, attributes, and aspects of God in the other person through your thought and feeling.

Prayer is an ever-present help in time of trouble; but you do not have to wait for trouble to make prayer an integral and constructive part of your life.

The sound basis for the art and science of true prayer is your knowledge and complete confidence that the movement of your conscious mind will gain a definite response from your subconscious mind, which is one with Boundless Wisdom and Infinite Power.

Effective prayer is based upon the spiritual premise that there is a Supreme Intelligence within us that becomes the thing we desire, to the degree that we accept this premise as being true. Then, as you give your attention in prayer to God and Truth, you create a state of consciousness that begins to express itself as *experience* in your life. If you maintain a sustained, affirmative attitude of mind, you will sooner or later reach a state of fulfillment, a sense of absolute conviction. The acid test of whether or not you have reached a conviction is when your mind accepts the idea completely and you can't conceive of the opposite. You must, in other words, unwaveringly believe in—accept as true—what you want. When you do, you will have truly impressed your subconscious mind, which must then respond accordingly. Then you know the answer will come.

▓

The scientific thinker knows that there are laws governing the operation of the entire cosmos and that, as Emerson says, "Nothing happens by chance. Everything is pushed from behind"—which means that if your prayer is answered, it is being answered according to the laws of your own mind, whether you are aware of it or not.

▓

Instead of mental striving, wrestling, or coercion, in scientific prayer you have Divine indifference. Divine indifference means that you know that it is impossible for your prayer to fail, in the same way you are absolutely positive that the sun will rise in the morning. You don't know how the answer will come, and you don't really care; you simply know the wisdom of your subconscious mind has ways of bringing about an answer to your prayer that your conscious mind does not know and could not even conceive of.

▓

Effective prayer demands forgiveness. As it is written, *And when ye stand praying, forgive.* (Mark 11:25)

You must eradicate hostility and resentment first, before you can pray successfully.

It is essential, in other words, that before you pray you eradicate all hostility and resentment and have love and goodwill for all men and women everywhere—as well as for the beasts of the field and everything else in the world. You must sense your essential unity with all things: the birds of the air, the fish of the sea, and indeed all growing things.

When praying, don't grit your teeth about it. Just know and claim that the joy of the Lord is flowing through you now, and wonders will happen as you pray this way.

Moreover, freedom and peace of mind will be yours as a result.

TYPES OF PRAYER

Praying to Let Go

In this prayer technique, you are not praying *for* some desired outcome to your concern or problem; instead, you release the source of your concern or problem to the Infinite Intelligence of your subconscious mind, which is the secret place from which we all draw forth the answers to all our problems. This is a powerful form of prayer when an individual or individuals are the source of your concern. To pray for them to change in accordance with your desired end would be interfering with their right to choose the lives they want. Instead, you relinquish your attachment to that person or those persons, and surrender them to God—knowing that in God there is guidance and right action. When we set others free and release them to God's guidance and direction, we are set free ourselves.

The Passing-Over Technique

This technique consists essentially in inducing the subconscious mind to take over your request as handed it by the conscious mind. As with all prayers, the passing-over technique is best accomplished in the reverie-like state, either immediately upon awakening or upon falling asleep. Know that in your deeper mind is Infinite Intelligence and Infinite Power. Next, calmly think over what you want, and then release it to your subconscious mind, seeing it coming into fruition from this moment forward. Be like the little girl who had a very bad cough and a sore throat. She declared firmly and repeatedly, "It is passing away now. It is passing away now." It passed away in about an hour. Use this technique with complete simplicity and naivete.

The Visualization (or Mental Movie) Technique

Your image of what you desire is the first cause relative to attaining the thing you are praying for.

In this prayer method, you quiet your mind and create a picture of yourself in your desired (prayed for) condition or circumstance, making that picture as vivid as you can, engaging all of your senses, knowing that what you form in your imagination is as real as any part of your body. In other words, just as what you see with the naked eye exists in the visible, external world, that which you can visualize in your mind's eye already exists in the invisible realms of your mind. That is why we say that any picture you hold in your mind believingly is *the substance of things hoped for and the evidence of things not seen.* (Hebrews 11:1)

The "Thank-You" Technique

In the Bible, Saint Paul recommends that we make known our requests with praise and thanksgiving. Some extraordinary results follow this simple method of prayer. The thankful heart is always close to the creative forces of the universe, causing countless blessings to flow toward it by the law of reciprocal relationship, based on a cosmic law of action and reaction.

For instance, what if your bills are piling up, you're out of work, and you have three children and no money. Regularly, every night and morning, in a relaxed, peaceful manner, repeat the words, "Thank you, Father, for my wealth," until the feeling or mood of thankfulness dominates your mind. Imagine that you are truly addressing the infinite power within you (knowing, of course, that you cannot see the Creative Intelligence or Infinite Mind). Realize that your thought-image of wealth is the first cause for obtaining your prosperity (or whatever it is that you desire).

If fear or thoughts of lack, poverty, and distress should come into your mind, say "Thank you, Father, for _____ [the condition you desire]" as often as necessary. As you keep up this thankful attitude, you will recondition your mind to the idea of whatever it is you desire, and your mind and heart will be lifted up to the point of acceptance.

The Argumentative Method

This method stems from the procedure of Dr. Phineas Parkhurst Quimby. Dr. Quimby, a pioneer in mental and spiritual healing, lived and practiced in Belfast, Maine, in the mid-nineteenth century. Quimby duplicated many of the healing miracles recorded in the Bible.

In brief, the argumentative method consists of spiritual reasoning whereby you convince yourself that the sickness is due to a false belief, groundless fears, and negative patterns lodged in your subconscious mind. You reason it out clearly in your mind and convince yourself that the disease or ailment is due only to a distorted, twisted pattern of thought that has taken form in your body. This wrong belief in some external power and external causes has now externalized itself as sickness. But changing your thought patterns can change it.

You explain to yourself that the basis of all healing is a change of belief. You also point out that the subconscious mind created the body and all its organs; therefore, it knows how to heal it, can heal it, and is doing so now as you speak. You argue in the courtroom of your mind that the disease is a shadow of the mind based on disease-soaked, morbid thought imagery. You continue to build up all the evidence you can muster on behalf of the healing power within, which created all the organs in the first place and which has a perfect pattern of every cell, nerve, and tissue within it.

Then, you render a verdict in favor of yourself and the healing of your problem. You liberate yourself by faith and spiritual understanding.

Your mental and spiritual evidence is overwhelming, because as you know that there is only one mind, what you feel as true you know will be resurrected in your experience.

The Absolute Method
When using the absolute method, you mention your name (or someone else's for whom you are praying), then your (or the other person's) unwanted circumstance, then you cease giving further thought to that circumstance by quietly and silently thinking of God and His qualities and attributes, such as, God is all bliss, boundless love, infinite intelligence, all-powerful, boundless wisdom, absolute harmony, indescribable beauty, and perfection. As you quietly think along these lines, you are lifted up in consciousness into a new spiritual wavelength, at which time you feel the infinite ocean of God's love dissolving everything unlike itself in your (or the other person's for whom you are praying) mind and body. You feel that all the power and love of God are now focused on you (or the other person), by immersing yourself in Infinite Intelligence, the consciousness of the Divine ideal, until you feel its presence within you. Whatever is bothering or vexing you (or the other person) is now completely neutralized in the presence of the infinite ocean of life and love, and your prayer will then be answered in ways mysterious and unknown to you and the other person.

The absolute method of prayer might be likened to sound wave or sonic therapy shown to me by a physician in Los Angeles. An ultrasound wave machine oscillates at a tremendous speed and sends sound waves to any area of the body to which it is directed. These sound waves can be controlled, achieving remarkable results in dissolving arthritic, calcareous deposits, as well as healing and removing other disturbing conditions.

To the degree that we rise in consciousness by contemplating qualities and attributes of God, we generate spiritual electronic waves of harmony, health, and peace.

The Decree Method

*T*hou shalt decree a thing, and it shall be established unto thee: and the light shall shine upon thy ways. (Job 22:28)

In this prayer method, you simply declare (decree) that what you are praying for is done. Remember that power goes into your word according to the feeling and faith behind it. You do not need to add power to power. In this prayer form, as in all prayer, there must be no mental striving, coercion, force, or mental wrestling. When you realize the Power that moves the world is moving on your behalf and is backing up your word, your confidence and assurance in this prayer will grow.

Examples of Prayer

Praying to Let Go

I knew of a man who operated a large market whose brother, a partner, had recently died. The brother had bequeathed a one-half interest in the business to his two nieces. The girls were very negative and demanding, creating all sorts of problems for this man. They refused to sell their one-half interest. The man told me that following an argument with them over their wanting more money from the business, he wrote down on a piece of paper, "I loose these girls to God completely. They are in their true place. Nothing is forever. This condition passes away *now*. It is God in action." He placed this writing in a drawer in his desk that was marked, "With God all things are possible," and forgot about it. In two weeks' time, his nieces agreed to sell their interest, and there was a perfectly harmonious solution.

A mother was distraught and highly agitated because her boy of eighteen had quit college and run away from home following an argument with his father. She was frantic, and her doctor had to prescribe strong sedatives to quiet her mind and body. In talking to her, I pointed out a few simple truths: You do not own your son; he came through you but not by you; Life-Principle is the common progenitor; we are all children of the one Father, or Self-Originating Spirit; your son is here to grow, to expand, and to overcome difficult challenges and problems, thereby enabling him to discover the powers within him and to release his talents to the world; you can't help him by mental excitation, anger, and resentment.

At my suggestion, she decided to release him completely. She decreed as follows: "I loose my son to God completely. He is Divinely guided in all his ways and Divine wisdom anoints his intellect. Divine law and order reign supreme in his life. He is guided to his true place and is expressing himself at his highest level. I loose him and let go."

She remained faithful to this prayer and daily claimed peace, harmony, joy, and Divine love for herself. Some weeks later, her son went back to college and began communicating with both parents, and his mother no longer feels possessive. She has discovered the riches of Divine love and freedom.

This woman ceased thinking from the standpoint of circumstances and conditions; she began to think from that interior stand-point where there are no circumstances, and from whence she was able to decree what conditions should be according to Divine law and order. Then she let the subconscious wisdom take care of the situation.

The Visualization (or Mental Movie) Technique

While on a vacation in Mexico, I met an attorney from Texas who told me that after this vacation, he had a very tough assignment before him in Dallas, concerning the settlement of conflicting claims among members of a family regarding a will involving about a million dollars. One member of the family had engaged him to bring peace and harmony so that a prolonged lawsuit could be avoided.

I suggested that he practice the following imaginative form of prayer therapy. Inasmuch as there is no time or space in the mental realm, he was to project himself mentally into a conference room in Dallas, where all the members of the family would be assem-bled. He was to claim that harmony, peace, and understanding were operating among them. Several times every day prior to this assignment, he was to imagine the member of the family who had hired him saying: "We have agreed to accept the terms of the will as written and will not contest it in court." He heard this over and over again and lulled himself to sleep every night with two words: "Happy ending."

Some weeks after I returned from the pyramids of Mexico, I received a letter from my attorney friend saying that he had fol-lowed my instructions, and that at the family conference there was a complete agreement and a happy ending.

The Decree Method

A young girl used the decree method on a young man who was constantly phoning her, pressing her for dates, and meeting her at her place of business. She found it very difficult to get rid of him. She decreed as follows: "I release _____ [the person's name] unto God. He is in his true place at all times. I am free, and he is free. I now decree that my words go forth into infinite mind and it brings it to pass. It is so." She said he vanished and she has never seen him since, adding, "It was as though the ground swallowed him up."

CORRECTING INCORRECT PRAYER

A widow once spoke with me about her need to sell an apartment building after her husband had passed on. She was in financial trouble, she had many vacancies, some tenants had not paid the rent, and the neighborhood was changing. She was afraid she would have to declare bankruptcy. The building was in the hands of brokers, but she had received no offers.

I explained to her that what she was seeking was also seeking her and that Infinite Intelligence within her would attract the right purchaser.

She prayed and also used her imaginative faculty and began to dramatize in her mind a buyer coming into her office, expressing an interest in her property. She imagined him saying to her, "I will buy it." She enacted this scenic dream several times a day, making sure that her mental imagery agreed with her affirmation of the truth. A few days after she began practicing this technique, a man came, looked the building over, seemed interested, but told her the next day that the price was too high.

The woman asked me to pray with her that this man would buy the apartment building. I explained to her that that would be the wrong approach and that she should never use mental coercion to force a sale, as that would be an invasion of the right of the buyer. I explained that Infinite Intelligence knows where the right buyer is and that that buyer would want and desire her building, that there was no acceptable occasion to *make* someone want it, and that she must realize that faith in the workings of her deeper mind would bring right results. We work by faith, not by hypnotizing others to do what we want.

As things turned out, the man who had rejected the building told his medical doctor about it, since this physician was looking for a good investment. The medical doctor bought the building and was delighted with the purchase. All the woman's problems were solved.

Mrs. B. had ulcers and was taking medicine prescribed by her doctors, but was nevertheless constantly saying, "The medicine is no good. My ulcers are worse." All her thoughts were of a bitter, ulcerated nature; she was resentful and full of hostility and suppressed rage toward relatives. She was at the same time petitioning a God far off up in the skies somewhere to heal her condition, which she unwittingly inflicted on herself. She was praying with a mind and heart full of hostility, suppressed rage, and resentment— which is praying amiss.

Ye ask, and receive not, because ye ask amiss. . . .
(James 4:3)

It was not until Mrs. B. replaced her hostility, rage, and resentment with divine love and peace that her prayers were answered.

Examples of Correct Prayer

Upon departing from a bus and arriving at her home, a lady discovered that she had lost a beautiful diamond ring and was quite perturbed for a while. She asked herself, "What is the truth about this ring?" She answered herself this way: "Nothing is lost in Infinite Mind. My subconscious mind knows where the ring is, and it leads me to it." After a few minutes she had the feeling that she should go back to the bus stop. She found the ring on the street close to the entrance to the bus.

To pray effectively, you change your mind to conform to the eternal truths of God, which never change. You do not beg, supplicate, or beseech. You simply reorder your mind and align yourself with the truth.

I had a conference with an ex-sergeant of the army who had served in Vietnam. He told me of a fascinating episode that had occurred during his tour of duty there. One afternoon when he was on patrol with his men, they walked right into six Vietcong soldiers, who immediately killed all five men in his patrol before they could lift their rifles. Obviously, the Vietcong had seen them coming and had ambushed them.

The enemy soldiers looked straight at him but never spoke to him or indicated that they saw him. They went through the pockets of his men and took papers, weapons, and all contents. He was amazed and could not understand it. He found his way back to his battalion and later wrote about his experience to his mother in Kentucky. She wrote back: "They did not see you, son. They could not see you or touch you, because I have prayed daily, 'My son will always be invisible to the enemy. God is his refuge and fortress.' "

This man's mother decreed constantly that her son would be invisible to the enemy and would be protected by God. This was communicated to her son's subconscious mind, which responded according to the impression or decree given. Every letter she wrote to her son concluded with these words taken from the 46th Psalm: "God shall help you, and that right early."

Undoubtedly these letters and prayers written by his mother had a profound effect upon him and made a deep impression in his subconscious mind, which responded to his mother's conviction of God's protection for him.

Effective Prayer Techniques

As you recite your prayers, let the impressions and feelings of the words sink into your deeper mind until your are possessed by their truth. As you continue this process, you will feel a great sense of inner release, like a cleansing of the soul. You will feel at peace and be relaxed, and you'll have a feeling that you are secreting the healing power from the depths of yourself that will bring about a perfect, harmonious solution to the desire you seek to resolve. That's when you'll know that your prayer is being answered.

There are four steps to praying effectively.

The *first* step is complete allegiance, devotion, and loyalty to the only presence and the only power—God. This Power is within you. It created your body, and It can heal it and all its problems.

Second, you must definitely, absolutely, and completely refuse to give power to any external thing or any other power but God. You give no power to the phenomenal world or to any person, place, or thing.

The *third* step: Whatever the problem, difficulty, or sickness may be, turn away from the problem and affirm knowingly:

"God is, and His healing presence flows through me now, healing, vitalizing, and energizing my whole being. God flows through me as the answer, as right action and Divine freedom."

The *fourth* step is to give thanks for the happy solution. Rejoice and say, "Father, I thank Thee for the perfect answer, and I know it is God in action now. I have mentally touched the power and the presence of God. It is wonderful!"

Principles to Remember and Apply

▶ Prayer is always the solution.

▶ Avoid all effort or mental coercion in prayer. Applying mental coercion or too much effort shows anxiety and fear, which block your answer. To use mental force is to presuppose that there is opposition.

▶ You delay the answer by thinking it will take a long time or that it is a major problem. Your subconscious has no problem; it knows only the answer.

▶ When you pray for another person, you are not sending a healing wave or thought-wave to that person. You are affirming that the Healing Love of God is in the subconscious of the other person.

▶ Praying is not begging or beseeching. To beg and beseech is to admit you don't have something, to attest to lack and limitation, which will inevitably attract more misery and loss.

▶ Refuse to take no for an answer. Believe implicitly in the promises of God.

❱ Prayer is aligning yourself with the eternal verities of life and becoming a focal point for the expression of life, love, truth, beauty, and the life more abundant.

❱ When you pray, it is essential that you be at peace with all people and things.

❱ Mentally act and feel the way you would act and feel were your prayer answered, and you will find that the power of faith will work wonders in your life.

❱ The four steps to effective prayer are: 1. Recognition of the Healing Presence; 2. Complete acceptance of the One Power; 3. Affirmation of the Truth; 4. Rejoicing and giving thanks for the answer.

❱ Divine indifference means that you know whatever you claim and feel to be true in your heart must come to pass, and you simply wait for the answer with great assurance.

5 The Healing Power of Forgiveness

Forgiveness is love in action. Without love in our hearts, we stumble and fall.

This is the acid test for knowing when you have forgiven the other: Suppose someone told you some wonderful news about the person who you say wronged you. How do you react? Do you resent it? Do you become disturbed? Would you rather hear the opposite? If so, you have not forgiven. The roots of anger and vengeance are still there.

You wither the roots through prayer and love.

You should rejoice to see the law of God work for anybody, regardless of who that person is, what he or she is, or where he or she is.

Forgive yourself by getting your thoughts in harmony with Divine Law and Order.

You cannot really forgive others completely until you have forgiven yourself first. To refuse to forgive yourself is nothing more or less than spiritual pride or ignorance.

※

Forgiveness of others is essential to mental peace and radiant health. You must forgive everyone who has ever hurt you if you want perfect health and happiness.

※

Your mind and forgiving heart must be in perfect alignment in order to get an answer to your prayers.

※

You do not get upset or resentful toward a person who suffers from a congenital deformity. Likewise, you should not be disturbed because some people suffer from mental deformities, that is, unkind, harsh, hurtful, cruel mentalities. Have compassion for them. Forgive them.

※

Be intolerant of false ideas, but not of people.

※

*A*nd if he trespass against thee . . . and . . . turn . . . to thee saying, I repent; thou shalt forgive him. (Luke 17:4)

To repent is to change your thinking along constructive lines and to keep it changed. Change how you are thinking, begin to *do justly, and to love mercy, and to walk humbly with thy God.* (Micah 6: 8), and you will have restored yourself to wholeness and will experience Divine forgiveness—which is the same as self-forgiveness, because The Source of All Forgiveness, God, is within you. You will feel the Divine Law of Love once again welling up and radiating through you, clearing away your self-condemnation.

If you steadfastly turn your thoughts God-ward, you cannot help but replace your feelings of self-recrimination with those of self-forgiveness, because in God there is only the principle of love, not of hate.

The law of forgiveness is a scientific law of mind. Think and act aright, and you will be forgiven, even if in the past you have not used the principles of mind to pursue the highest good for yourself and others.

Perfunctory, mechanical mouthing of prayer won't accomplish forgiveness. Only when a real inner transformation takes place and you possess a hunger and thirst to do the right thing, then this seeming miracle of forgiveness for past errors takes place and you discover that a new beginning is a new end.

*T*hen came Peter to him, and said, Lord, how oft shall my brother sin against me, and I forgive him? till seven times? Jesus said unto him, I say not unto thee, Until seven times: but, Until seventy times seven. (Matthew 18:21-22)

The only way to wither unforgiveness is with love—by wishing for the other person all the blessings of life, until you can meet the person in your mind, and you can sincerely react with a benediction of peace and goodwill. This is the meaning of *forgive until seventy times seven.*

There is no time or space in the mind-principle. The minute you decide to transform your life by filling your subconscious with life-giving patterns, the Infinite Healing Presence cleanses your subconscious and you become free.

The Life-Principle never condemns or punishes you. You punish yourself by misuse of the law and by negative or false thinking.

The marvelous and wonderful truth is that you have the power to forgive and stop disparaging yourself for your shortcomings and mistakes by deciding to change your thoughts and keep them changed. On the basis of scientific mental law—which is that your subconscious mind automatically accepts any thought held believingly—the moment you begin to think constructively, harmoniously, peacefully, and lovingly, based on eternal truths that never change, your subconscious will immediately respond to your constructive thoughts and imagery, the past will be forgotten and remembered no more.

It makes no difference what wrongdoing you have committed. The law of your subconscious does not hold any grudge against you. Once you have made a sincere decision to become a transformed person and to practice and live the eternal truths of God, "thou art made whole."

Forgiveness of yourself and others makes way in your mind for the Infinite Healing Presence to flow through you.

All our derelictions, sins, errors, crimes, hostilities, and resentments are wiped out when we change our hearts and acknowledge that the love and harmony of God reign supreme in our lives.

When Divine Love, Divine Harmony, and Divine Peace dominate your mind and heart, the law of your subconscious, being compulsive, will compel you to express the qualities and attributes of God. Your old ways will be as if they never were, the "old" you will be no more; all your new ways will be ways of pleasantness, and all your paths will lead to peace.

Self-condemnation brings failure and misery. Self-forgiveness brings happiness, peace, and triumphant living.

Forgive yourself and learn to accept forgiveness.

You are a son or daughter of the Infinite. Have a healthy, reverent, wholesome respect for the Divinity that created you and watches over you, and that created the whole universe and all things contained therein. Make a habit of exalting the Divine Presence within you and then living accordingly.

⬛

The past is only your memory of the past. The results of past events—be they good or bad—are still but the expression of your present thinking. The only pain and sting you can experience is the pain of the present moment. Think of peace, harmony, joy, love, and goodwill in this moment. By mentally dwelling on these things and claiming them, *and forgetting the past*, a new and glorious life will be yours. You are a good person *now*; that's all that matters. The past is dead. Nothing matters but this moment. You are a good person now, and you have a perfect right to all the blessings of life now. *Remember ye not the former things, neither consider the things of old.* (Isaiah 43:18)

⬛

God condemns no one. He has already forgiven you. Now forgive yourself. Change your thought and keep it changed. Think on whatsoever things are true, just, noble, and of good report. Think from the standpoint of the Golden Rule and the Law of Love.

⬛

Here's a parable about forgiveness:

> A little boy had been very bad. His mother gave him a lot of chores and tasks to do about the house and kept him indoors for a week. He fulfilled all the tasks joyously, and at the end of the week his mother said, "You are a very good boy. Your work is excellent."
>
> The little boy replied, "Mother, am I not just as good now as if I never had been bad?"
>
> His mother answered, "Of course you are! How wonderful is the truth!"

Cling to the good, the beautiful, and the true, and you will experience forgiveness, for you will have become just as good now as if you had never been bad.

※

You pass judgment on yourself by the concepts and beliefs that you entertain. You are always choosing your thoughts, and in that act you are passing judgment on yourself. God, however, sees you as perfect. The Perfect One cannot see imperfection.

※

Forgiveness is giving to the other love, peace, and all the blessings of life. As you give, you are blessed, as *It is more blessed to give than to receive.* (Acts 20:35)

※

You forgive yourself when you identify mentally and emotionally with the ideal of good, and you continue to do so until it gels within you as a conviction or subjective embodiment.

Let God's love enter your soul. If you resolve to be a new person in God, then the past will be wiped out and remembered no more.

You sin when you think negatively and resent, hate, condemn, or engage in fear or worry. And you are always sinning when you deviate or turn away from your announced goal or aim in life, which should always be peace, harmony, wisdom, and perfect health: the life more abundant.

To sin is to miss the mark, which is the goal of health, happiness, and peace.

Your sins will be canceled by forgiving yourself—by turning your attention back toward the aims of peace, harmony, wisdom, and perfect health—*and* when you forgive those against whom you hold resentment and hate.

Forgiveness is getting your thoughts in line with the Divine Law of Harmony.

Resentment, condemnation, remorse, and hostility are behind a host of maladies. There is only one remedy: Discard your hurts. The one and only sure way to do this is by forgiveness.

⬛

The Bible says, *Love ye one another*. Anyone can do this who really wants to. Love means that you wish for the other health, happiness, peace, joy, and all the blessings of life. For that, there is only one prerequisite: the *willingness* to forgive, which must then be accompained by sincerity.

⬛

To forgive the other does not necessarily mean that you like that other person or want to associate with that person. It simply means that you wish for the other what you wish for yourself.

⬛

Another way of understanding *forgive until seventy times seven* is that your life should be dominated by a constant attitude of forgiving, or giving for. Continue supplanting negative thoughts with constructive, harmonious thoughts, and you will be constantly forgiving yourself.

Remember, too, that your thoughts about another are also your thoughts about yourself. You are the only thinker in your world, and your thought is definitely creative. You and you alone are responsible for the way you think. Whatever you think or wish for another you are creating in your own body, experiences, conditions, and events.

It behooves you, therefore, to forgive.

⬛

Your subconscious never sleeps. It is always on the job, even as *you* sleep. Forgive yourself and everyone else before you go to sleep, impress your subconscious with forgiveness thoughts, and the healing of any kind that you desire in your life will take place much more rapidly.

Let us suppose you had a painful abscess on your jaw a year ago, and you told me about it, and I asked you if you had any pain now. You would say, "No. I have a memory of it, but no pain."

Now let's say I were then to tell you something wonderful about someone who had wronged you, cheated you, or defrauded you, and you felt gladness at hearing the good news about this person. Clearly, you have a memory of the old pain, but not the sting in your heart. You have truly forgiven.

Dwell on these wonderful words: *But if the wicked will turn from all his sins that he hath committed, and keep all my statutes, and do that which is lawful and right . . . all his transgressions that he hath committed, they shall not be mentioned unto him: in his righteousness that he hath done he shall live.* (Ezekiel 18:21–22)

You are told in these verses that if you will begin to practice right thinking, right feeling, and right action, you will have made yourself a new person. The old you will then be forgiven and re-membered no more.

THEY ACCEPTED THE HEALING POWER OF FORGIVENESS

A woman came to see me stating that she was a Christian and her husband was of another faith. They were quite happy together until she began receiving letters from her mother saying that she had done great evil, letters that contained religious threats plus moral condemnation. I explained to this woman that in God there is no Greek or Jew, no bond or free, no Christian or Muslim, no Hindu or atheist. God has no religion and knows nothing about creeds, dogmas, and human opinions.

I then told her the story of a spiritual teacher who taught his students as follows: "Compose a letter written as from a friend to yourself that would completely satisfy you if you received it. Put into exact words what you would like your friend to write or say to you."

Every night, this woman embraced her mother in her imagination and radiated love, peace, and joy to her; then she would read to herself the imaginary letter from her mother that filled her soul with joy. She continued to do this every night for about three weeks. At the end of that time, she received a letter from her mother apologizing for her previous letters and containing almost the exact words the woman had been picturing, feeling, and rejoicing in each night.

This is the great law of substitution or forgiving: substituting love and goodwill for any feeling of ill will or hostility. You can practice this same technique with anyone with whom you are having difficulty.

A man who murdered his brother in Europe visited me many years ago. He was suffering from great mental anguish and torture, believing that God must punish him. He explained that his brother had been having an affair with his wife, and that he had shot him on the spur of the moment. Since that incident, this man had married an American woman and had been blessed with three lovely children. He held a position in which he helped many people, and he was a transformed man.

My explanation to him was that he was not the same man who shot his brother. Mentally and spiritually he was a new man. He was now full of love and goodwill for humanity. The "old" man who committed the crime many years before was mentally and spiritually no more. This man was actually condemning an innocent man!

This explanation had a profound effect upon him, and he said it was as if a great weight had been lifted from his mind.

Doreen B. was raised by an aunt and uncle after her parents were killed in an accident. She told me that she had never recovered from the abuse she suffered at their hands. "It still haunts me," she said. "I wake up every day asking myself how anyone could torment a little kid that way. No matter how hard I tried, I was punished for making a mess, for making noise, for not doing my chores fast enough or well enough. It was awful!" She continued after a moment, "And do you know what's really terrible? They convinced me. Whenever anything goes wrong for me, right away I think, 'I must have deserved this.' Hard as I try, I can't forgive myself for not being perfect."

I explained to Doreen that forgiving herself meant extending that same forgiveness to those who had harmed her.

I then taught her a simple but effective method to bring about forgiveness in herself. "Think of God and His love for you," I told her. "Quiet your mind, relax, and let go. Then affirm this prayer."

I fully and freely forgive [think of the name of the offender].
I release him or her mentally and spiritually. I completely
forgive everything connected with the matter in question. I
am free, and he or she is free. It is a marvelous feeling.
This is my day of general amnesty. I release anybody and
everybody who has ever hurt me, and I wish for each and
every one health, happiness, peace, and all the blessings of
life. I do this freely, joyously, and lovingly.

I then told her: "Whenever you think of the person or persons
who hurt you, say, 'I have released you, and all the blessings of life
are yours.' You will then be free and they will be free."

As Doreen discovered, the great secret of true forgiveness is
that once you have forgiven a person, it is unnecessary to repeat
the prayer. After a few days, thoughts of the person or experience
will return less and less often, until they fade into nothingness.

Forgiveness Techniques

Many people are full of guilt because they failed to visit a loved
one prior to that person's death. Their statements are somewhat as
follows: "I mistreated my mother before she passed on"; "My husband died, and I was out at the time"; "I did not forgive my father,
and now he is dead and gone."

The first thing you must realize is that there is no time or
space in the Mind Principle. This very moment you can relax mentally and think of the person whom you believe you wronged in
some way. Imagine that you are talking with that person. Exalt that
person in your mind, and tell the person of your love for him or
her; realize that the Presence of God is there and that His love,
light, truth, and beauty are flowing through you and the other person. Live in this imaginary scene. Continue to dramatize this mental scene until you get a reaction that fills your soul with joy and

sets you free. The action of God will then have taken place, and a complete healing within you will follow.

▨

This may be the most powerful forgiveness prayer you can utter:

I forgive _____ [person's name], for he or she (or you can repeat the person's name) knows not what he or she does.

Principles to Remember and Apply

▶ You know when you have forgiven another, because you can meet the person in your mind and there is memory of the pain but no longer any sting.

▶ To *forgive* is to sincerely wish for the other what you wish for yourself: harmony, health, peace, and all the blessings of life.

▶ Forget the past and saturate your mind with Divine love, peace, and harmony. No matter what has happened in the past, you can change it now.

▶ Fill your subconscious with life-giving patterns of thought and you will erase and crowd out everything unlike God, and forgiveness will be yours.

▶ It is necessary to enter into the spirit of forgiveness and goodwill in order to get real and lasting healing.

▶ Forgive yourself if you feel you have wronged someone who is deceased. Exalt that person in your mind. Feel the Presence of God there; realize that. His light, love, truth, and beauty are flowing through you and that person.

▶ Perfunctory prayer won't accomplish forgiveness. Only when a real inner transformation takes place and you possess a hunger and thirst to do the right thing will this seeming miracle of forgiveness take place.

❯ *Forgive until seventy times seven* means your life should be dominated by a constant attitude of forgiving. Continue supplanting negative thoughts with constructive, harmonious thoughts and you will be constantly forgiving yourself and others.

❯ All our shortcomings are completely forgiven when we become dominated by Divine love, harmony, and peace; then the law of our subconscious responds accordingly. And because the law of our minds is compulsive, our old patterns will be no more, and our new ways will be ways of pleasantness and paths of peace.

❯ To forgive means to give forth love, goodwill, harmony, and all the blessings of life on all people.

❯ The Life Principle is forever forgiving and healing you.

❯ Forgiveness opens the way for the Infinite Healing Presence to flow through you. Criticism, resentment, and hostility to others all block the Healing Presence.

6 The Mysterious Power of Desire

*Let your desire captivate and hold your attention,
knowing that what you are seeking is seeking you.*

■

The Infinite Power that gives you the desire will also reveal to you the perfect plan for its fulfillment.

■

In order to make your will the will of Omnipotence, you must animate it. You must make your will alive within you by enthusiasm, until it becomes embodied in the subconscious mind. This is called desire.

■

What things soever ye desire, when ye pray believe that ye receive them, and ye shall have them. (Mark 11:24)

In these few cryptic words is the specific and motivating direction for making use of the creative power of thought and bringing forth our desires.

You must understand that for anything to have substance in the realm of mind, it must be *actually existing there*: Your thought, or desire, in other words, is as real on its own plane as your hand or your heart.

Following the Biblical instruction, once you give thought to your desire with conviction, you completely eliminate from your mind all consideration of conditions, circumstances, or anything that might imply adverse contingencies. *You pray believing that you have already received it.* Have faith in the reality of your desire, and you will attract everything necessary for its fulfillment. You are planting a seed in your mind by impressing upon the subconscious the particular thing that you desire. If you leave it undisturbed, it will infallibly germinate into external fruition.

The mere fact that you have a desire for which you seek an answer means that the answer is already present in your mental and spiritual world.

You must give before you can get. You must put the seed in the ground to get a harvest. Likewise, in order to feel the joy of the fulfilled desire, you must let the Universal Energy flow through your ideals, hopes, and aspirations—your desires—vitalizing and energizing them.

You must appreciate the fact that your desire—the new play, book, script, trip, enterprise, or adventure—is already real in your mind, though invisible. To know that what you desire is real, that it has form, shape, and substance on the mental plane, gives you scientific faith. This knowledge enables you to pass through doubt, worry, and uncertainty to a place of conviction deep in your subconscious mind, knowing that whatever desire you believingly convey to your subconscious will be projected on the screen of space and will reach fruition.

When you pray for your desire, you aren't giving vitality to it; vitality is already inherent within it. What you're doing is nourishing its manifestation as form, function, experience, or event.

When you want something, do not think of all the reasons why you can't have it, but realize there is an Infinite Intelligence that will attract to you what you want. As you accept this truth, the deeper currents of your mind will bring it to pass.

If you don't believe that you have *the right* to your heart's desire, you won't be able to believe that you *will have* your desire.

Practice the law of silence. When you have a desire, don't discuss it with anyone except when it is absolutely necessary to do so—as, for example, someone who is directly involved. You can share it with a spiritual advisor, who is there to aid you. To talk with anyone else—friends, relatives—however, can prove to be unwise, as often they will ridicule your desires and diminish your faith in attaining them successfully.

The less you talk about your ideal, the better. Keep on nourishing your goal with faith and confidence, and when you have established the mental equivalent, its success will burst forth like a flower in full bloom.

A desire is a prayer. The desires of an atheist can be answered just as well as those of any religious person, as long as the atheist puts his or her whole faith into the desires. The law of mind, like the laws of nature, works for one and all.

Whatever you desire is already available as a thought in your mind. Claim what you want and feel its reality, remembering that Infinite Mind is spaceless and timeless. Cease limiting yourself, therefore, by postponing your desires because of your conscious mind's concerns about your present circumstances. Remind yourself that external events, conditions, and circumstances are not causes. Remove all stumbling blocks that are in your mind and enter now into the joy of the answered prayer.

Your desire is reminding you of something in your life that, if accepted by you and is in accordance with the eternal verities, will make your life fuller and happier. Don't postpone it. You can realize in your mind the desire of your heart without procrastination. *Hope deferred maketh the heart sick . . .* (Proverbs 13:12)

You have to plant the seed before you can reap; you have to give before you can get. Give the Universal Source of Supply (God)—the Power, Cause, and Substance of all things—your attention and loyalty. Then pour energy, life, love, and attention on that which you want. When you have succeeded in establishing the mental equivalent in your mind, the result will follow.

*D*elight thyself also in the Lord; and he shall give thee the desires of thine heart. (Psalm 37:4)

When you desire something and your conscious mind is of the belief that some other person is necessary for the fulfillment of your desire, you must not try to make that other person bend to your will through use of any subtle mental influence of prayer or by envisioning the person acting in accordance with your will or desire. You must trust the Infinite Intelligence of your subconscious to attract to you the right person at the right time and in the right way. It makes no mistakes. Trust the infinite intelligence to bring your desires to pass; then there is no occasion for mental coercion or trying to influence others to do your bidding.

When you sense your oneness with your desire, Infinite Intelligence moves on your behalf and brings your desire to pass. This is the creative law operating in you. Such knowledge works wonders in your life.

※

You can bring your desire to pass without hurting a hair of a living being in this world. As Saint Paul said, *Love is the fulfilling of the law.* (Romans 13:10)—not coveting, dominating, or the like. When you think right, feel right, act right, and do right, you have used the law constructively—and your desire will come to pass and there will be goodwill toward and for all.

※

Envy of another will sabotage the attainment of your goals. You don't have to want anything that some other person is enjoying. God's infinite riches are available to all.

※

Ralph Waldo Emerson said, "Nothing was ever achieved without enthusiasm." Therefore, you must back your desire with enthusiasm.

※

Desire is an absorbing or controlling possession of the mind by an interest or pursuit.

※

Do not let yourself be led astray from your desire by negative beliefs, doubts, fears, worries, or the opinions of others.

The fear thought that challenges your desire must die, and

your desire must live. Take your attention completely away from the thought of opposition; this will starve the opposition thought to death. Feast mentally and emotionally on your ideals and goals in life.

Your loyalty, devotion, and attention must be given to your goal, ideal, or desire.

God is within you, and your desire to achieve is from God. God gave you your brain, your mind, the hands to write and build, and the urge to achieve and express, plus the intelligence and capacity to do all these things.

Open your mind and heart to the realization that God who gave you your desires will also reveal to you the perfect way for their manifestation. You must believe in your heart and accept the reality of your desire in your mind. Be thankful for its fulfillment. In spite of appearances, conditions, or circumstances, you must know that the Living Spirit will respond, creating the fulfillment of your dreams.

You must feel your idea or desire as true. Then, when it is accepted subconsciously, your conscious wish or desire will have passed from mere wishing and desiring to a subconscious conviction, and your subconscious will bring it to pass. The law of the subconscious is one of compulsion, and the will of the subconscious comes to pass.

Only when you turn your desires over to your subconscious with certainty will they come to fruition.

The greater the expected benefit from the desire, the stronger is the desire. Where there is no expected benefit, gain, or advancement accruing, there is no true desire; consequently, no action is found working toward the manifestation of the desire.

Failure over a long period of time to listen to your desires to be, to do, and to have will lead to frustration and unhappiness. Extinction of desire means apathy, no feeling, and no action.

Desire is the moving principle of universe. It is creative power and must be channeled and directed wisely.

Affirmations and prayer will not change matters. What is essential is that these are imbued with a strong desire. It is *this* combination that has the power to bring into your life prosperity of all kinds.

Realize that as Shakespeare said, "All things be ready if the mind be so." This means that you must order your mind and thoughts to conform to the age-old truth that whatever you are seeking already exists in Infinite Mind. All you have to do is identify mentally and emotionally with your desire, realizing that it is as real as your hand or heart.

Desire is the Life Principle seeking to express Itself at higher levels through you. It is the angel of God, the messenger of the Divine, saying to each one of us, "Come on up higher." Your desire is Life seeking to manifest Itself in some form through you, which as yet exists only as thought-image in your mind.

Your desire is your prayer; prayer is the soul's sincere desire.

Many people indulge in fantasizing about something pleasant while nevertheless believing it could never happen to them, because they think that what they desire for themselves is too good to be true. This is a pure waste of time and results in debilitating one's entire mentality. Go all the way with your idea! Don't say, "Oh, that's too good to be true." Say, rather, "I welcome this idea! I accept it wholeheartedly and it will come to pass in God's good time." You must realize that there is nothing too good to be true, and nothing too wonderful to last.

*B*elieve that ye receive them, and ye shall have them.
(Mark 11:24)

A young man asked Socrates how he could obtain wisdom. Socrates replied, "Come with me." He took the lad to a river, pushed the boy's head under the water, held it there until the boy was gasping for air, then relaxed and released his head. When the boy regained his composure, Socrates asked him, "What did you desire most when you were under water?"

"I wanted air," said the boy.

Socrates said to him, "When you want wisdom as much as you wanted air when you were immersed in the water, you will receive it."

In a like way, when you really have the desire to overcome any block in your life and you come to a clear-cut decision that there is a way out and nothing will divert you, then what you desire will be yours.

Be careful that your desires do not conflict with your beliefs, your imaginings.

Emile Coue, the famous psychologist from France who visited America in the early part of the twentieth century, defined the law of reversed effort as follows: "When your desires and imagination are in conflict, your imagination invariably gains the day."

If, for example, you were asked to walk a plank on the floor, you would do so without question. But suppose the same plank were placed twenty feet up in the air between two buildings. Would you walk it? Your desire to walk it would be counteracted by your imagination, or fear of falling. Your dominant idea, which would be the picture of falling, would conquer. Your desire or will to walk on the plank would be reversed, and the dominant idea of failure would be reinforced.

No one can serve two masters. You cannot expect to realize the desire of your heart if you believe there is a power that thwarts that desire. If there were some power to challenge God, God would cease to be omnipotent or supreme. Learn to believe that the Infinite Intelligence that gave you the desire will also show you how to fulfill it.

Your desire to dance is God seeking to reveal to you that this is a universe of dancing forces. The whole world is a dance of God.

Your desire to paint a sunset is the indescribable beauty of God seeking expression through you, the artist.

God gave you ears to hear the music of the spheres and His still, small voice within, which ever says to you, *This is the way, walk ye in.*

God gave you eyes that you might see God in everything.

Your desires are the Infinite revealing His riches to you and saying to you *thou art ever with me, and all that I have is thine.* (Luke 15:31)

DESIRE FULFILLED THEIR LONGINGS

Here's a letter I once received.

Dear Dr. Murphy:

My eighth birthday was approaching and my mother asked me what gift I would treasure most. I spent most of my spare time doing woodcraft and had been given many good ideas by carpenters building a house nearby, including the reverence for a Disston saw made of very fine steel and superior craftsmanship. So I told her of my burning desire for one, since it would improve my work.

Wishing to surprise me, Mother started on her sleuthing trips, first to hardware stores, then to secondhand stores, but the answers to her query were almost a stereotype: "Impossible—you'll not find one; they have not been made since the war!"

Feeling very downcast, Mother told me of her exhaustive search and said that, since the Disston saw was impossible to find, I must choose another gift. I told her that it was not necessary for the saw to come from her or the hardware store, but that I knew the saw would come.

We had had our home up for sale, had a buyer with a deposit in escrow, and had one termite inspection in which the inspector had examined only the house and basement, but the buyers wanted a double-check by another company, which is not generally done. The second inspector was much more thorough and insisted on examining the attic. After about an hour he returned to the living room with a beautiful old saw with a hand-carved handle. Engraved across one side in flourishing letters was the word *Disston*. I later learned that when the house had been built, one of the carpenters had lost it in a very narrow aperture between the framework for a large skylight in the living room and the stonework of the back of a large fireplace.

I have always been grateful that you taught me at an early age to understand and to contact the all-knowing Power within me.

Your friend, R. Conrad.

I once performed a marriage ceremony for a young secretary who told me that about six months prior to her marriage, she had drawn up a treasure map for herself, dividing it into four parts. In the first section, she wrote, "I give thanks for God's wealth flowing freely in my life." In the second, she wrote, "I give thanks for a four-month tour around the world." In the third, she wrote, "I give thanks for a wonderful, spiritual-minded man who harmonizes with me perfectly." In the last, she wrote, "I give thanks for a wonderful home that is beautifully furnished." Underneath these four requests, she wrote, "I give thanks for the immediate fulfillment of all these requests in Divine order through Divine love."

Every morning, afternoon, and evening, she would go over her requests, affirming and imagining their fulfillment, realizing that gradually these images would be written in her subconscious mind, which would bring them to pass.

The answer to her first request came in about a month's time. Her grandmother in New York bequeathed $50,000 to her in her will, along with a new luxury car. Her mother and father, who were living in Canada, invited her to take a trip with them around the world, and on the trip she met a young scientist. As she said, it was love at first sight, and her marriage to him took place on her return to California. He had a beautiful home, magnificently furnished.

She said to me that writing out a treasure map and trusting the infinite intelligence of her subconscious mind really worked. And it does.

Techniques for Harnessing the Power of Desire

Twice a day, quiet the activity of your mind and remove all tension from your body by simply talking to it and telling it to relax. This brings about an outcropping of your subconscious mind, and all effort and negative thoughts will be reduced to a minimum. Know that if you order it in this way, it has to obey. In that quiet, receptive, peaceful state, focus your attention completely on your desire. *Feel* the joy and reality of it all. Become identified with the picture of your desire in your mind, and have faith that what you *imagine* and *believe* must come to pass. Think, imagine, speak, and act the way you would if you possessed your desire. For example, if you wanted a beautiful home, picture that ideal home in your mind—imagine yourself walking through the house, watering the garden, and playing with the children. Make it vivid and real. Feel its naturalness. Feel the solidity of the walls and the furniture. Show your friends through the house. Live there mentally, and what you imagine and feel to be true will come to pass. Then, turn this request over to your subconscious mind, releasing it with absolute faith and confidence in the same way that a farmer deposits a seed in the ground, trusting implicitly in the laws of growth, knowing that your subconscious will likewise respond according to the nature of your request.

Affirm often: I believe that the subconscious power that gave me this desire is now fulfilling it through me.

Principles to Remember and Apply

▶   Nothing is accomplished without desire.

▶   Picture the fulfillment of your desire and feel its reality. Identify mentally and emotionally with your desire and walk in the assumption that your prayer is answered.

▶   Accept that God who gave you the desire will bring it to pass in Divine order. There is no power to oppose Omnipotence.

▶   The answer to the desire of your heart depends on the intensity of your imagination, backed up by the realization that Infinite Intelligence will move on your behalf, bringing it to pass in Divine order.

▶   Desire is the cause of all feeling and action, and it is the moving principle of the universe.

‣ Place all of your attention on only what you desire, and you will begin to reconcile the opposition in your mind.

‣ You must put the foundation of desire under your goals.

‣ You must not try to make another bend to the will of your desire through the use of prayer or by envisioning the person acting in accordance with your will or desire. This would be an invasion of the other person's rights. Trust the infinite intelligence to bring your desires to pass as it deems best.

‣ The Life Principle will flow through you rhythmically and harmoniously if you consciously affirm: "I believe that the subconscious power that gave me this desire is now fulfilling it through me."

‣ The desire and the imagination must agree. When your desire and your imagination are in conflict, your imagination always wins.

‣ Dismissing your desire as something that can't come to pass because it is too good to be true is a waste of time. Remember, there is nothing too good to be true, nothing too wonderful to last for the Infinite Intelligence within you.

7

The Persuasive Power of Gratitude

Express thanks now for your blessings.

◼

*T*his is the law of thanksgiving: A grateful heart is always close to God. As you give thanks daily for your health, abundance, security, and many blessings, God multiplies your good exceedingly. This is based on the law of action and reaction, which is cosmic and universal.

◼

Express thanks *now* for your blessings and to those whose friendship and kindness and support have blessed you.

◼

A poet once said: "Oh, God, give me one more thing—a grateful heart."

◼

The whole process of acquiring mental, spiritual, and material riches may be summed up in one word: *gratitude*.

※

A grateful thought for any good received is in itself a prayer from the heart, and blesses you.

※

Have you ever had the experience of wanting to purchase something—a book, an item of clothing, or even a car—and found it out of stock? If the salesperson told you he or she would order it and deliver it, *you were absolutely sure of receiving the item you desired in the near future, exactly as you requested, because you believed in the salesperson.*

How much more should you trust and believe in the Infinite and His creative law, which never changes and which responds with absolute fidelity to your trust and belief in It!

※

Praise and gratitude do not move God or the Law, but they *do* bring about a transformation in our minds and hearts so that we become a spiritual and mental magnet, attracting all kinds of good from countless sources.

※

Your gratitude, your praise, and your measure of thankfulness must not be expressed as a fawning attitude seeking favors. It must be a rejoicing that all things you need and claim are within you, waiting for you to receive them with a joyful and thankful heart.

You are truly grateful and have a heart full of praise when you become aware of and appreciate the universal principles of life and the Providence that gave you everything from the foundation of time.

Gratitude keeps you in tune with the Infinite and connected with the creative law. The value of gratitude, however, does not consist purely in drawing to you many blessings. You must remember that without the thankful heart, you become dissatisfied with your present condition and circumstances.

The grateful person is one who continually and invariably expects the good things of life. This person's expectation inevitably takes material form. The creative law of your subconscious mind, in other words, makes you into the image and likeness of that which you contemplate.

A man complained to me that a person he saved from drowning did not even thank him or offer him a reward, even though he had risked his life in order to save the man. I explained to him that he had done the right thing and that Life would reward him, but that he must not look to a particular person to reward or to thank him. Your good does not always return to you from the source where you expended your effort or money.

THE POWER OF GRATITUDE WORKED WONDERS FOR THEM

A young man named Lucien Hamilton Tyng was born in Peoria, Illinois, which offered very little for the ambitions of this young man, for he dreamed big dreams and thought expansively. Lucien decided to go to Chicago and try his luck. He got a job as an office boy, which barely paid him a living wage. After his room rent was paid, it left him exactly fifty cents a day for meals. He found that a five-cent bag of chocolate cream made a very filling lunch. Breakfast was fifteen cents, so dinner could not be more than thirty-five cents. Lucien was very religious, and he made it a constant habit to hold his fifty-cent piece in his hand and say: "God multiplies this and I give thanks. I am receiving more and more money every day." He would repeat this for about ten minutes every morning, before he spent the fifty cents. He began to attract many clever and successful men, and opportunities began to arrive his way that he was quick to take advantage of. "Thank you, Father," was constantly on his lips.

As the years passed, many influential men began to seek his opinion and were guided by it. He seemed to be miraculously gifted, and his mental acumen gradually increased. Other men admired his sagacity in business and he was deeply trusted. He solved many business problems for them. Before and after every successful achievement, his constant prayer was, "Thank you, Father."

One day a wonderful idea came to him, which he related to a good friend who said it had tremendous potentialities. They formed a partnership and incorporated what was then called the General Gas and Electric Company. It grew by leaps and bounds, with stations all over the eastern states. After many years, they sold the company for a reported sum of fifty million dollars.

A Realtor I know named Rick W. proved that a thankful attitude improves every department of your life, your health and happiness as well as your prosperity.

Rick had been having a great deal of difficulty selling homes and properties that were listed with him. He was frustrated and unhappy. Convinced of the prosperity power of the grateful heart, however, he began to pray every night, affirming as follows: "Father, I thank thee that thou hast heard me, and I know that thou hearest me always." Then, just prior to sleep, he condensed the phrase to two words: "Thank you." He repeated them over and over again, as a lullaby; he continued to speak these two words silently until he fell asleep.

One morning a woman came into Rick's office whose face Rick was sure he recognized. He prided himself on his memory for names and faces, but when she introduced herself, the name meant nothing at all to him. At that moment, he realized that he had seen her in a dream a night or two earlier. While he was still pondering this amazing fact, she told him that she represented a consortium that was actively investing in rental properties. By the end of the day, Rick had sold her group more properties than he had sold over the previous month.

A maid was putting aside a few dollars a week out of her meager wages in order to buy a car. Her sister gave her a copy of one of my books, *The Power of Your Subconscious Mind*, and she read it avidly. She later told my secretary that she sat down one night and wrote a letter to herself in order to impress her subconscious mind with the idea of a car. The gist of her letter was that she gave thanks to God for the lovely car that she now had and that she accepted it gladly and rejoiced that it was fully paid for and functioning perfectly. She placed the letter in a desk drawer and marked the envelope, "My answered prayer. Thank you, Father."

The sequel is interesting. On the following Sunday she went to her church and, during a conversation with one of the ushers, she commented on his new and beautiful Cadillac. He said, "I want to sell one of my cars. Do you know anyone who wants a good car?" She replied, "I do, but I have only $450 saved." The usher said, "That will be all right; I have no storage space for it. Take the car for $450"—which she did.

She had figured it would take her about three years to accumulate funds for a down payment on a car. But in expressing gratitude, she had claimed the car *now*.

A man said, "Bills are piling up, I have no money, and I must go into bankruptcy. What shall I do?" I suggested that for ten or fifteen minutes, two or three times a day, he sit down quietly and affirm boldly, "Thank you, Father, for thy riches now," and to continue in that relaxed and peaceful manner until the feeling or mood of thankfulness dominated his mind.

I told him that as he kept up this grateful attitude, he would recondition his mind to the idea of wealth—and that is exactly what happened. He subsequently met a former employer at a social gathering who offered him an executive position and also advanced him a considerable sum of money, which enabled him to pay off all his bills and be free of debt.

I received a letter from a businesswoman in Chicago named Jessica R. Her son Kevin, who was eight, had been ill for about a year with chronic asthma. He often had paroxysmal attacks that sent him to the emergency room.

One night, Jessica sat by her son's bedside after he went to sleep and prayed out loud:

> Kevin, you are God's son. I see the Presence of God in you now. This is the presence of harmony, health, peace, joy, vitality, and wholeness. God breathed into you the breath of life. The Spirit of God made you, and I know the breath of the Almighty gave you life. You inhale the peace of God, and you exhale the love of God. *Father, I thank thee that thou hast heard me. And I knew that thou hearest me always.* (John 11:41–42)

Jessica prayed in this way for about an hour, reiterating these great truths and knowing that they would sink into the subconscious of her son. At a certain point, she felt a sense of inner peace that her prayer was answered, and she had no desire to go on praying any longer.

When Kevin woke up in the morning, he said, "Mommy, last night an angel came to me and said I don't have to have asthma any more. Isn't that awesome?" In the days and weeks that followed, it became clear that the asthma really was gone. The child had completely recovered.

Techniques for Harnessing the Power of Gratitude

There is a law of gratitude to which you must conform in order to get wondrous results in your life.

> *First,* you accept completely and wholeheartedly that there is an Infinite Intelligence from which all things flow.

> *Second,* you believe that this Source responds to the nature of your thought.

Third, you relate yourself to this Infinite Intelligence by a deep feeling of inner gratitude.

Silently decree the following words morning, night, and throughout the day: "Thank you." *Feel* the reality of your expression within. You are thanking your Higher Self for abundance, health, wealth, and harmony.

Principles to Remember and Apply

▶ Take time every day to quiet your mind and affirm: "Thank you, Father, for Thy riches now." Lull yourself to sleep with "Thank you" on your lips. Give thanks for what you now possess and for your many blessings. Count these one by one and God will multiply your good exceedingly.

▶ Many people contribute to your well-being. Include them in your prayer of gratitude. This will bring you into subconscious communication with the good in all people and in everything—and the riches of life, the earth, and all people will gravitate automatically toward you.

▶ The attainment of mental, spiritual, and material richness may be summed up in one word: *gratitude*.

▶ Give constant praise and be thankful for your knowledge of the creative laws that can bring all you desire to you.

▶ Gratitude keeps you in tune with the Infinite and connected with the creative forces of the universe, and you become a mental and spiritual magnet attracting countless blessings.

▶ Show your deep appreciation for those around you, members of your family, and your coworkers. People crave appreciation. Give it freely and lovingly.

) If you have only a dollar in your pocket, bless it by saying, "God multiplies this money exceedingly in my experience and I am grateful for the constantly increasing, tireless flow of God's riches in life." You will attract fantastic wealth.

8 The Boundless Power of Imagination and Visualization

Your imagination is the treasure-house of infinity. It releases from your subconscious mind all the precious jewels of music, art, poetry, and invention.

▧

The fulfillment of your desire depends upon the intensity of your imagination, not upon the presence of any particular external conditions or facts.

▧

Imagination is the action of forming mental images or concepts of what is not actually present to the senses. This is why it is said that where the five-sense person sees an acorn, the person with imagination sees an oak tree.

▧

Ask yourself, "What am I visualizing now in my personal, professional, and romantic life? Is it only for my good, or is it also what others in my life would wish for themselves?" The mental picture to which you remain faithful will be developed in your subconscious mind and consequently be made manifest in your experience.

※

Your image of what you desire is the first cause relative to attaining the thing you are praying for.

※

Your mental patterns and images are made manifest by your emotional attachment. Whatever idea or desire you emotionalize and feel as true is accepted unequivocally by your subconscious and made manifest in your world.

※

Your outer world and all its happenings, experiences, and events are projections of your inner mental images. When you become conscious of the distinction between your inner, causal world of imagination and the outer world of effects, you begin to truly understand how to bring your desires to fulfillment.

※

Before anything can be created, it must be imagined. That is why the language of imagination is the language of God. In the beginning, Infinite Intelligence brought forth all things in the universe through creative imagination . . . *so God created man in his own image, in the image of God created he him; male and female he created them.* (Genesis 1:27)

Infinite Intelligence started the idea for a world by envisioning a sun, moon, stars, and all things contained in this limitless cosmos. All Its dreams come to pass. The Infinite Source of All becomes the thing It imagines Itself to be.

This same vitality of Divine imagination is in you.

Identify yourself now with your goal by mentally and emotionally uniting with it. Energize your ideal in your mind by frequently visioning its fulfillment. As you persevere and remain faithful to your vision, Infinite Energy will flow through your mental pattern and cause your desire to cross over from the mental image to subconscious embodiment.

Whatever you imagine and *feel* as true, *will* and *must* come to pass—even though the evidence of the five senses seems to deny it.

You can liken your conscious mind to a camera and your subconscious mind to the sensitive plate on which you register and impress pictures. Your mental pictures are developed in the darkroom of the subconscious mind.

When you are able to imagine the reality of a fulfilled desire and feel the thrill of accomplishment, your subconscious will bring about the realization of your desire.

Imagination is one of our most powerful faculties; it is the treasure-house of infinity. Disciplined, controlled, and directed imagination is a mighty instrument that plumbs the depths of your subconscious mind, bringing forth new inventions, discoveries, poems, and music. Scientists, artists, musicians, physicists, inventors, poets, and writers draw forth riches from the treasure-houses of their imaginations and bless humanity in countless ways.

You can discipline, control, and direct your imagination constructively and get what you want in life, or you can use it negatively by imagining the fears and worries that you don't want.

When the world says, "It is impossible, it can't be done," the person with a vivid imagination says, "It *is* done!"

It is just as easy—and far more interesting, captivating, and alluring—for you to imagine yourself to be rich and successful as it is to dwell on poverty, penury, and failure. If you wish to bring about the realization of your desires or ideals, form a mental picture of fulfillment in your mind; constantly imagine the reality of your desire. In this way, you will actually bring it into being.

What you imagine as true thereby already exists in your mind; if you remain faithful to your ideal, it will one day objectify itself. The Master Architect within you will project on the screen of visibility that which you impress on your mind.

Mental images that you consciously accept as true are impressed on your subconscious mind and made manifest in your life. This was proved by Dr. Hans Selye at the University of Montreal's Institute of Experimental Medicine and Surgery, who demonstrated that the subconscious mind does not differentiate between stress states caused by *imagined* worries and stress states caused by *real* concerns. Dr. Selye showed that if a person persists in indulging in imagined worries, the body will create excess hormones that will play havoc with the body, causing psychosomatic disease.

Remember, then, that the law of your mind is that you will get a reaction or response from your subconscious mind according to the nature of the thought or idea you hold in your conscious mind. The subconscious will not argue with you. If you *negatively* discipline, control, and direct your imagination by imagining fears and worries, that is what you will bring into your life. Or you can *constructively* discipline, control, and direct your imagination and get what you want in life and according to your belief it will be done unto you.

Unless there is first an image in the mind, it cannot move, for there would be nothing for it to move toward. Your prayer, which is your mental act, must be accepted as an image in your mind before the power from your subconscious will play upon it and make it productive.

▦

With your disciplined imagination, you can soar above all appearances, discord, and sense evidence, and imagine the way things ought to be, realizing the sublime principle of harmony operating through, in, and behind all things.

▦

Every picture that you create in your mind, particularly when emotionalized, comes to pass. It works out in action, either internally or externally. If you inhibit it from working out in external action, it is inevitable that it will manifest itself in some mental, physical, or emotional disharmony in the body.

▦

As you are visualizing your desire, will discover that there will come a time when you no longer feel driven to do so. This is the sure psychological sign that you have embodied your desire subjectively. It has become an inner knowing. Having realized your desire subjectively, you will have no further compulsion to pray for it.

THE POWER OF IMAGINATION AND VISUALIZATION CHANGED THEIR LIVES

Dr. Lothar von Blenk-Schmidt, a member of the Rocket Society and an outstanding research electronic engineer, gives the following condensed summary of how he used his subconscious mind and imagination to free himself from certain death at the hands of brutal guards in a Russian prison camp coal mine. He states as follows:

"I was a prisoner of war in a coal mine in Russia, and I saw men dying all around me in that prison compound. We were watched over by brutal guards, arrogant officers, and sharp, fast-thinking commissars. After a short medical checkup, a quota of coal was assigned to each person. My quota was three hundred pounds per day. In case any man did not fill his quota, his small food ration was cut down, and in a short time he was resting in the cemetery.

"I started concentrating on my escape. I knew that my subconscious mind would somehow find a way. My home in Germany was destroyed, my family wiped out; all my friends and former associates either were killed in the war or were in labor camps. I said to my subconscious mind, 'I want to go to Los Angeles, and you will find the way.' I had seen pictures of Los Angeles and I remembered some of the boulevards and buildings very well.

"Every day and night I would imagine I was walking down Wiltshire Boulevard with an American girl whom I met in Berlin prior to the war. In my imagination we would visit the stores, ride buses, and eat in the restaurants. Every night I made it a special point to drive my imaginary American automobile up and down the boulevards of Los Angeles. I made all this vivid and real. These pictures in my mind were as real and as natural to me as one of the trees outside the prison camp.

"Every morning the chief guard would count the prisoners as they were lined up. He would call out, 'One, two, three,' and so on. [One morning,] when number seventeen was called out, which was my number in sequence, I stepped aside. [At that moment,] the guard was called away for a minute or so, and on his return he started by mistake on the next man as number seventeen. When the crew returned in the evening, the number of men was the same, and I was not missed, and the discovery of the error would take a long time.

"I walked out of the camp undetected and kept walking for twenty-four hours, resting in a deserted town the next day. I was able to live by fishing and killing some wildlife. I found coal trains going to Poland and traveled on them by night, until finally I reached Poland. With the help of kind strangers, I made my way to Lucerne, Switzerland.

"One evening at the Palace Hotel in Lucerne, I had a talk with a man and his wife from the United States. This man asked me if I would care to be a guest at his home in Santa Monica, California. I accepted, and when I arrived in Los Angeles, I found that their chauffeur drove me along Wiltshire Boulevard and many other boulevards that I had imagined so vividly in the long months in the Russian coal mines. I recognized the buildings that I had seen in my mind so often. I had reached my goal."

Indeed, there are marvelous wonders in the subconscious mind! The American girl whom von Blenk-Schmidt had met in Berlin before the war and had imagined, in the prison camp, walking through Los Angeles with, did, in fact, become his wife!

In an article in *Everybody's Magazine*, Henry M. Flagler, the Standard Oil multimillionaire, stated that the master secret of his success and his immense wealth was his capacity to image a thing as a finished form. In other words, he imagined the end, the final result, and all the forces of the Infinite Intelligence came to his aid. He actually *envisioned* the whole project as completed. He disciplined, controlled, and directed the image in his mind.

If he knew there was oil in a certain area, for example, he would close his eyes and imagine the train tracks on the ground, the trains running and steaming, the derricks, and the men going to work, talking and laughing. He heard the train whistles blowing and saw the steam. He imagined the whole scene with a remarkable sensory vividness, feeling the reality of the finished project until it became natural to him. Then, having impregnated his subconscious mind, he found that all the forces of the Infinite came to his aid. By the law of attraction, he was provided everything he needed for the fulfillment of his dream.

During a series of lectures in Kimberley, South Africa, I met a most interesting man; I told him I would refer to him in my writings. He was a soldier in the Second World War, and his leg was severely wounded by gunfire. He was on crutches in an English hospital for a long time.

He began to think, saying to himself, "There is an Intelligence which made me; It can heal my leg." He began to picture himself doing all the things he would do were he whole and perfect. Having been an athlete before the war, he lived the life of an athlete in his mind, maintaining a picture of himself as he wanted to be. He participated in the mental movie, dramatized it, felt it, and made it real. He said he was unable to walk, but in his chair he would *feel* himself riding a bicycle, climbing mountains, or kicking a football. Furthermore, he began to claim he was strong and powerful.

The amazing result of this was that in a few years his leg healed perfectly where the major bones were broken. He was once again able to compete in athletic competition, with a great many successes.

A schoolteacher who listened to my daily radio program wrote to me, saying that she had written in a notebook the words *Health, Wealth, Love,* and *Expression.* She said that she lacked health and sufficient money, was unmarried, and was seeking an opportunity to teach in a college.

Under *Health* she wrote in her notebook: "I am all health; God is my health."

Under *Wealth,* she wrote: "God's riches are mine now, and I am wealthy."

Under *Love,* she wrote: "I am happily married and Divinely happy."

Under *Expression,* she wrote: "Divine intelligence guides me to my right work, which I perform in a perfect way for a wonderful income."

Every morning and evening, she would look at what she written in her book, and claim: "All these desires are now being fulfilled by my subconscious mind." She would then take some time to picture the complete result under each category. She would imagine her physician saying to her, "You are completely healed. You are all right now." She would imagine her mother, with whom she lived, saying to her, "You are rich, now. We can move and travel. I'm so happy." She would then imagine a minister saying, "I now pronounce you man and wife," and she would "feel" the naturalness, solidity, and tangibility of an imaginary ring being placed on her finger. Prior to sleep, her last mental picture was of her principal saying, "Sorry you are leaving, but I am glad to hear of your college assignment. Congratulations!"

She would run each mental movie separately for about five minutes in a completely relaxed and joyous manner, knowing that these pictures would sink down into her deeper mind, where they would gestate in the darkness and be made manifest at the right time in the right way. Within three months' time, all her desires were fulfilled.

Techniques for Applying the Power of Visualization and Imagination

Goethe, the great German philosopher and writer, used his imagination wisely. He was accustomed to filling many hours quietly holding imaginary conversations. His custom was to imagine one of his friends sitting before him in a chair, answering him in the right way. In other words, if he were concerned over any problems, he imagined his friend giving him the right or appropriate answer, accompanied by the usual gestures and tonal qualities of the voice, and he made the entire imaginary scene as real and as vivid as possible.

Practice mental imagery prior to sleep. Make a real mental movie of your desired aim, dramatizing it to the best of your ability, and knowing that your subconscious mind is the receptive plate on which your conscious imagery will be impressed.

In the science of imagination, you must first begin to discipline your imagination and not let it run riot. You must eliminate all the mental impurities, such as envy, covetousness, fear, worry, and jealousy. You must remember that fears do not exist save in your imagination turned morbid. Failure will never come to pass unless you keep up a morbid picture charged with the emotion of fear. If you constantly indulge in such a mental picture, of course, you will bring failure to pass, because even though you have the choice of failure or success, you are choosing failure.

Focus all your attention on your goals and objectives in life and refuse to be swerved from your purpose or aim, which is to lead a rich and happy life. Become mentally absorbed in the reality of your desires.

Enthrone now in your mind the mental images, ideas, and thoughts that heal, bless, enrich, inspire, and strengthen you, and you will see them take material form in your world. It is true that you become what you imagine yourself to be.

Your sustained imagination is sufficient to remake your world. It is the *sustained* mental picture that is developed in the depth of the mind.

Trust the laws of your mind to bring your good to pass, and you will experience all the blessings and riches of life.

Principles to Remember and Apply

▶ Imagination is one of the foremost faculties of your mind. When disciplined, it enables you to realize your ideas, dreams, or aspirations and project them on the screen of space.

▶ Project a mental movie in your mind night and morning, knowing that your conscious mind is the camera, and it will be developed in the darkroom of your subconscious mind.

▶ Imagine the happy ending or solution to your problem, feel the thrill of accomplishment, and what you imagine and feel will be accepted by your subconscious mind and bring it to pass.

▶ In mental imagery, you must *feel* the picture to vitalize it.

▶ As you imagine an objective clearly, you will be provided with the necessities to achieve it through your subconscious mind.

> The truths you accept consciously must be emotionalized and felt as true to be assimilated by your subconscious mind.

> Infinite Intelligence's ways are past finding out. Imagine the end and your subconscious will bring it to pass in ways you do not understand.

9

The Magical Power of Silence and Serenity

The quiet mind receives the answer.

▦

Real power comes from inner quiet. The quiet mind gets things done.

▦

The deepest desire of every person is peace of mind; the pursuit of any and all desires is ultimately for peace of mind.

▦

Thomas Carlyle said, "Silence is the element in which great things fashion themselves."

▦

The secret of outstanding achievement is in developing what is called the "quiet mind."

Confucius said: "The superior man is always quiet and calm."

You can achieve a balanced life in which serenity and tranquillity reign supreme. The key is to acquire mental and emotional control.

To know peace, cease completely talking about your ailments and your worries and anxieties about world conditions, for that will only magnify your inner troubles and make your condition worse, because your mind always amplifies what it looks upon.

Periodic withdrawal during the day from sense evidence and the noise and confusion of everyday living carries with it all the benefits of sleep—that is, you become asleep to the world of the senses and alive to the wisdom and power of your subconscious mind.

There can be no inner peace until all the sorrow, hates, grudges, and vindictiveness are expunged from your mind and heart.

If you really want peace of mind and inner calm, you will get it. Regardless of how unjustly you have been treated, or how unfair the boss has been, or what a mean scoundrel someone has proved to be, all this makes no difference to you when you awaken to your mental and spiritual powers. You know what you want, and you will definitely refuse to let the thieves (thoughts) of hatred, anger, hostility, and ill will rob you of peace, harmony, health, and happiness. You cease to become upset by people, conditions, news, and events when you identify your thoughts immediately with *your* aim in life. Your aim is peace, health, inspiration, harmony, and abundance. Feel a river of peace flowing through you now. Your thought is your invisible power, and you can choose to let it bless, inspire, and give you peace—and move you into the life you desire.

Emerson said, "Let us be silent that we may hear the whispers of the gods."

God is peace and is at the very center of your being.

Emerson said, "Nothing can bring you peace but the triumph of principles." Choose to live your life by the principles of God, and the peace that passeth all understanding will be yours: There is a principle of beauty, but none of ugliness; there is a principle of harmony, but none of discord; there is a principle of love, but none of hatred; there is a principle of joy, but none of sadness; there is a principle of opulence and abundance, but none of deprivation and poverty; and there is a principle of right action, but none of wrong action.

The secret of abiding peace of mind is to become identified with the Infinite Presence and Power within you, which is ineffable peace. As this inner peace comes to you, you unite mentally and emotionally with the Infinite Presence within you of love, harmony, and power, feeling these qualities flowing through you.

An aviator knows that if he or she flies right into the center of a great hurricane or cyclone, there is stillness and calm. Likewise, in the midst of the storms of your life dwells God (Life Principle, Cosmic Consciousness, Infinite Intelligence)—absolute peace. Direct yourself mentally and emotionally into the secret dwelling place of Infinite Peace within you, and like the aviator flying into the heart of the cyclone, you will find yourself in the place of calm.

Energy, power, inspiration, guidance, and wisdom come out of the silence and the stillness of the mind when tuned in with God.

Many people take tranquilizers to give them a certain sense of peace and relaxation. Drugs, even though they may give you a sense of well-being for a time, do not bring about a change of mental attitude, which is essential. Pills to stimulate or pills to depress are not the answer to anxiety, excess tension, or worry. It is spiritually misguided to drug ourselves so that we become insensate to the stresses or anxieties of living. We are here to meet the challenges, difficulties, problems, stresses, and strains of life, so that in the process we may discover the fulfilling life through our great source of peace: the Divinity within.

※

We create our own tensions, anxieties, and high blood pressure by the way we react mentally and emotionally to people, conditions, and events. It is of the utmost importance, therefore, to keep constantly in mind that the power is in you and not in others. Externals are the effects, not the cause. You have the ability to attain *the peace of God, which passeth all understanding* amid the commotion of the world. Other people or conditions may *suggest* certain things to you, but *you are the only thinker in your universe,* and you can refuse to accept any harmful, unsettling suggestions of any nature whatsoever.

A realization of the presence and power of God in you and of your capacity in thought to tune in to the Divine Power will enable you to bring peace, harmony, and divine order into your life.

※

The way to be *en rapport* with the Infinite Intelligence within— your subconscious mind—is to be relaxed, peaceful, and confident.

※

Come back to the center within yourself where God abides. Here all is peace, bliss, harmony, and joy. Here you live beyond time and space. Here you are alone with God. You are in the sacred center. You are invulnerable, and all the negation of the world cannot touch you.

HOW THE POWER OF SILENCE AND SERENITY STRENGTHENED THEM

A woman once said to me that she spent a half hour in the Silence every day but got no results in achieving communion with the Divine Presence. I discovered that her procedure was to listen to music, have incense burning, and focus her attention on statues of holy men. She also adopted certain postures, lit candles, erected altars in her home, and faced the East when she prayed. She was completely involved in the periphery; her mind was focused on statues, candles, rituals, incense, music, and postures. She was impregnating her mind with the sensations of her five senses and was not in fact communing with the Divine Presence at all. Practice turning away from the world and the evidence of your senses. As Longfellow said: "Let us then labor for an inward stillness—a stillness and an inward healing—that perfect silence where the lips and the heart are still and we no longer entertain our own imperfect thoughts and vain opinions, but where God alone speaks in us and we wait in singleness of heart that we may know His will and in the *Silence* of our spirit that we do His will and do that only."

Checking into a hotel in Madrid, I joined the line moving slowly toward the registration desk. I overheard the clerk trying to pacify a very angry, irate woman. She called him stupid and a fool, and said that he should be discharged.

It was interesting to see his reaction. He replied, "I am sorry, madam. There must be some mistake. Your name is not registered with us, and there is no reservation according to our records. I will do the best I can and will certainly find something for you."

She went into a strident tirade, punctuated at intervals by the clerk's, "Yes, madam," and, "I'm very sorry about it all, and if I were on your side of the desk, I should feel just as you do."

I observed this young man. There was no angry retort. No color came to his cheeks; he revealed no annoyance or irritation. He looked calmly and dispassionately at the woman and was friendly, pleasant, courteous, and quite efficient.

When I reached the desk, I said to him, "I admire your composure. You are to be complimented." Then he quoted a text, verse 19 of the twenty-first chapter of Luke: *In patience possess ye your soul.*

He did not allow the tirade of the woman to ruffle him. He was master of his thoughts and responses.

I once attended a religious convention at Airlie, near Washington, D.C., where I spoke on the topic, "Law Which Never Changes." During the five days I was there, I had a long talk with a very successful and immensely wealthy man, who told me that the secret of his health, wealth, and outstanding achievement was in the developing of what he called the "quiet mind."

He had a card in his pocket on which the following great truths were inscribed:

"The superior man is always quiet and calm." (Confucius)

In quietness and in confidence shall be your strength. (Isaiah 30: 15).

He that is slow to anger is better than the mighty, and he that ruleth his spirit than he that taketh a city. (Proverbs 16:32)

The Lord thy God shall bless thee in all thine increase, and in all the works of thine hands, therefore thou shalt surely rejoice. (Deuteronomy 16:15)

Except the Lord build the house, they labour in vain that build it. (Psalm 127:1)

This man said that every morning of his life, he anchored his mind on these truths, repeating them slowly, quietly, and lovingly, knowing that as they were impressed in his subconscious mind, he would be compelled to express success, health, vitality, and new creative ideas. He has established four large corporations and is advisor to many executives in different fields. He travels the world over.

He said to me, while presenting me with one of his meditation cards, which he dispenses freely, that thirty years ago he met a man on a ship to Europe who explained to him that if he took certain constructive words from the Bible—words that represent the eternal truths of God and His Law—his mind would become anchored on the Supreme Presence, which responds as you call upon It.

The whole key to his riches was that he knew as he meditated on the bible phrases regularly, systematically, and repetitiously, that he was activating the latent power within his subliminal depths, compelling him to move onward, upward, and God-ward.

Another prominent businessman I once had the pleasure of meeting told me that he attributed all his successful business decisions to fifteen-minute silent periods in the mornings. He withdrew his attention and sensory awareness from the external world, quieted his body, closed his eyes, and contemplated the great truth that Infinite Intelligence is within him. Silently, he affirmed that God was guiding him; that new, creative ideas were given to him; that the Divine Presence would govern the conferences of the day; that God thought, spoke, and acted through him; that the right words were given to him by the Supreme Wisdom within him; and that all decisions for his company were based on right action.

He then spent about five minutes in meditation, imagining God's peace flowing through his whole being. Often, while in this quiet period, solutions to acute business and personnel problems popped into his mind, problems that he and other associates had been struggling with for days.

He stated he had discovered that the quickest way to get an answer to a problem was to turn over the request to that center of quietness, knowing the answer would emerge.

Techniques for Capturing the Power of Serenity and Silence

For ten or fifteen minutes every day, sit quietly; relax; let go; empty out all hate, ill will, and self-condemnation; fill your soul with God's love; and affirm: God's love fills my mind and heart, and I pour forth love and goodwill to all those around me and all people everywhere. If I have a grudge or a feeling of ill will toward any particular person, I single him or her out in my mind and pour out blessings upon him or her until I meet him or her in my mind and there is no longer any sting.

▨

Practice speaking, acting, and responding from the Divine Center within you. Before you go off on a mental debauch or explosion, say, "God in me thinks, speaks, acts, and responds to all of life." This will still your mind.

▨

Let go, relax, and still the wheels of your thought processes. Speak to your subconscious mind with gentle authority and conviction, telling it to take over in peace, harmony, and Divine Order, and it will conform to your command. You will find that all the functions of your body will become normal again.

When you go to a well, pond, or fountain for water, you take a bucket or some other proper receptacle in which to receive the water. In the same manner, go to the Infinite as if you were going to a pond, with your receptacle being your receptive mind. It will be filled with the Infinite Healing Presence and all the gifts of God. Silently dwell on the presence of God within you. Go into His Presence with a receptive and expectant attitude, knowing that Infinite Intelligence will respond when you call.

Before you go to sleep, turn away from the concerns and worries of the day and give your attention to the great principles and truths of life. Think about the great, the wonderful, and the good. Refuse to describe or even talk about the trials and troubles of the world. Your anxieties and worries will diminish and you will develop a quiet mind in a troubled world. Let the peace of God rule in your heart.

Principles to Remember and Apply

▶ All the powers of God are within you, waiting to be drawn forth by your conscious mind when it is stilled.

▶ Peace will come to you when you realize that God, who gave you the desire for health, happiness, abundance, and security, can bring all your dreams to pass in Divine Order.

▶ The quiet mind gets things done. The wisdom of your subconscious rises to your surface mind, or conscious mind, when it is relaxed and at peace. It is then that your subconscious goes to work to execute the idea of your conscious mind.

▶ Nothing can bring you ultimate peace but the triumph of a life lived in accordance with Divine principles.

▶ You can't find inner peace until you empty your mind of all hate, ill will, and self-condemnation.

▶ You achieve inner peace by filling your soul with God's love, and by understanding that events, conditions, and circumstances are effects and that the cause is in your own thought and feeling. Fill your mind with the thoughts of love and goodwill to all. This mental attitude will give you peace and harmony.

▶ To attain peace, learn to let go. Quiet your mind, immobilize your attention, and realize that God alone knows the answer.

▶ There are creative answers in your subconscious; the answer will come in Divine Order, and the day will break for you and all the shadows will flee away.

10 The Creative Power of Sleep and Dreams

*Your subconscious, in its dream nature, is revealing
to you the nature of the impressions you have
made upon it, pointing out to you the course your
life is taking.*

■

Your subjective mind performs its highest functions when your
objective senses are in the state of abeyance called sleep. The best
time, therefore, to impregnate your subconscious with your
thoughts of good, your prayers for healing of body or circumstance,
your determination to change, and the like is prior to sleep: Your
conscious mind is submerged to a great extent when in a sleepy
state, and you avoid the conflict between your desires and your
imagination.

■

The highest degree of outcropping of the subconscious occurs
prior to sleep and just after we awaken. In this state, negative
thoughts that tend to neutralize your desire and so prevent acceptance by your subconscious mind are no longer present.

Often our conscious minds get involved with the vexations, strife, and contentions of the day, and it is necessary to withdraw from the objective world and commune silently with the inner wisdom of our subconscious minds. Is this not prayer? Is this not what occurs during sleep? Sleep, thus, can be thought of as a form of prayer.

Remember that your subconscious mind is impersonal and nonselective—it will accept your negative, resentful, or hateful thoughts as well as the good thoughts, and will act accordingly. The subconscious also magnifies and multiplies whatever you deposit in it, *good or bad*. Hence, be mindful of the thoughts and feelings you go to bed with. The thoughts and feelings you have prior to sleep are transmitted to your subconscious mind, which then begins to act on them as though they were your request or desire for guidance. Before you drift off to sleep, cleanse your mind of all disturbing, vexatious thoughts of any kind, thus creating a clear channel for the Divine energies to flow through you constructively as you sleep.

Dr. John Bigelow, a famous research authority on sleep, demonstrated that at night while asleep, you receive impressions showing that the nerves of the eyes, ears, nose, and taste buds are active, and also that the nerves of your brain are quite active. He says that the main reason we sleep is that during sleep, "the nobler part of the soul is united by abstraction to our higher nature and becomes a participant in the wisdom and foreknowledge of the gods."

Research analyses of dreams show that the symbols appearing in the individual subconscious apply to each individual only. The same symbols appearing in two different dreams, or in the dream of a friend or other member of your family, will most likely have very different meanings. For example, Joseph's interpretations of the dreams of Pharaoh could only have applied to Pharaoh.

Self-preservation is the first law of life, and your subconscious always seeks to protect and preserve you from harm of every kind. One means it uses to do this is dreams.

You may, therefore, at times have a precognitive dream accompanied by a deep intuitive feeling of impending danger for yourself or a loved one. If your dream presages an unhappy or tragic occurrence relating to yourself or someone close to you, do not deride it as a mere fabrication of your imagination or as a harmless hallucination. Listen to it. Your subconscious is always trying to warn you of any impending condition of harm in time for you to avoid it.

More often than not, the imagery in our dreams is symbolic, but we can train ourselves to dream literally. For several years I have been suggesting to my subconscious prior to sleep, "I dream literally and clearly, and I remember my dream." Over a period of time, I have convinced my subconscious mind of this truth, and as a result, close to 90 percent of my dreams are literal in the same way you read your morning newspaper. In this way, I also receive many answers to my prayers in dreams.

※

At times a dream may cause you to question some prevailing belief, thought, or action you are holding. Infinite Intelligence, in other words, often uses the occasion of sleep to stir us up, create a quarrel in our minds, and challenge our false indoctrinations, creeds or dogmas, compelling us instead to listen to God and Love.

※

Generally speaking, when a certain dream occurs repeatedly night after night—either in the same form or some variation—your subconscious is dramatizing it because it is very important to you. The way to distinguish these dreams from those that have no real import or substance for you is that typically you cannot trace the source of these significant dreams to some recurring activity you are engaged in immediately prior to sleep (such as reading an impressionable fear-inspiring horror or murder imply novel or true crime story).

※

All your dreams are dramatizations of your subconscious and in many instances they warn you of impending danger. All dreams suggestive of a negative eventuality in your life, however, can be changed, and none is fatalistic.

There is no such thing as inexorable fate.

Remember, you are the master of your own destiny. You mold, fashion, and shape your own future by your *thought and feeling,* not by your dreams. Anything in your subconscious is subject to change, and when you know the laws of mind, you can create or recreate your future.

▓

When you dream, your conscious mind is asleep and is creatively joined to your subconscious, which then dramatizes its contents in the form of dreams.

▓

Robert Louis Stevenson devotes a whole chapter of *Across the Plains* to dreams. He was a vivid dreamer and had the persistent habit of giving specific instructions to his subconscious every night prior to sleep. He would request his subconscious to evolve stories for him while he slept. If Stevenson's funds were at a low ebb, his command to his subconscious would be something like this: "Give me a good, thrilling novel that will be marketable and profitable." His subconscious responded magnificently.

▓

The last waking concept you have before going to sleep is often etched into your subconscious mind. At times, your subconscious will dramatize the thought when your conscious and subconscious are creatively joined in sleep. This can be the cause of pleasant or unpleasant dreams, depending on the nature of the thought you had before you drifted off to sleep.

▓

It is commonly accepted that sleep is intended for rest of the body. But your subconscious mind and the processes of your body, though slowed down considerably, continue to function. A deeper reason why we sleep is to develop spiritually. The Divinity that shapes our ends is All-Wise and has so arranged it that we are compelled to withdraw from the world of noise, which is not conducive to unfoldment. In sleep, therefore, we are often Divinely guided.

THE POWER OF SLEEP AND DREAMS GUIDED THEM

A man apparently in perfect health dreamed on several occasions that he was being operated on for a disorder of the prostate gland. He asked me if I thought he should see a doctor for a checkup but stated that he had no symptoms or pain of any kind. I clarified the workings of his subconscious mind to some degree; namely, that it seeks to protect him at all costs. I suggested that he should see his physician immediately and get a complete checkup by a urologist. However, he deferred seeing his doctor. In a few days' time he developed a urinary constriction and blockage and was in excruciating pain. His physician took him to the hospital and had a skilled urologist operate on him immediately. I visited him in the hospital shortly after that and he remarked to me, "I should have paid more attention to my dream and acted sooner." However, I am happy to say he made a wonderful recovery, as he continued to fill his subconscious mind with thoughts of wholeness, harmony, vitality, and perfect health.

You will perceive that his subconscious mind was actually warning him to do something, as it knew of the prostatic infection and enlargement. The foreshadowing idea, the presentiment that he was going to be operated on, was probably caused by the already existing condition. He had made an error in delaying a medical examination.

The words of the ancient proverb are true: "Night [sleep]

brings counsel." The key to its practical application can be developed through your continual awareness.

※

At a dinner at the house of friends in Los Angeles, I got to talking with a young woman named Colleen M. When she mentioned that she was in computer graphics, I said, "That's a very active field these days, isn't it?"

"It certainly is," she replied. "A little too active sometimes! As a matter of fact, I just had to deal with a really difficult problem. An Internet-related company in New York offered me a job. It would have meant a good deal more money than I'm getting where I am, but of course I would have had to move to New York."

"How did you decide what to do?" I asked, intrigued.

"I went off to one of my favorite spots, up in the hills, and quieted my mind," she replied. "Then, I asked myself, 'How would I be feeling right now if I had just made the right decision about this?'"

"And what did yourself answer?" I asked.

She smiled. "Myself told me I would feel wonderful. I would be happy and confident about my decision."

Act as though I am, and I will be. Colleen had discovered this truth in her own life. She acted as though she had made the right decision, knowing that the creative Principle of Life is one of love and responsiveness and that it loved her and cared for her. She began to say, "Isn't it wonderful! Isn't it wonderful!" over and over again. That night, she lulled herself to sleep with the feeling, "It is wonderful."

That night she had a dream. She was back at her favorite spot, gazing off toward the distant coastline. Suddenly she realized that the wind in the bushes was speaking words. It said, "Stand still!

Stand still!" She woke up. She knew that she had just heard the inner voice of intuition.

"What did you do?" I inquired.

"The only thing I *could* do," she told me. "I listened to my inner voice. I turned down the New York offer. And it's a very good thing I did. You may not believe this, but I heard today that the firm just let go about thirty percent of its people. If I'd moved there, I might be out of a job now."

I once had a telephone call from a woman in New York City, stating that her husband had told her that he planned to take a large sum of money from his private safe and invest it in a foreign country for greater returns. A few days later he passed on, and when the safe deposit box in the bank was opened, there was no cash, but there was a record at the bank that two days previously he had visited the vault. There was no trace or record of any investment, and a minute inspection of his desk revealed no clues.

I suggested to her that she turn her request over to her subconscious mind, which knew the answer, and that it would reveal the answer to her in its own way. She prayed as follows prior to sleep: "My subconscious knows where my husband secreted that money, and I accept the answer and believe implicitly the solution will come clearly into my conscious mind." She quietly dwelled on the meaning of these words, knowing they would be impressed on her subconscious, thereby activating its response.

She had a very vivid dream in which she saw a small, black box hidden behind a picture of Lincoln on the wall in her husband's work den. She was shown in the dream how to press a secret button, which could not be seen with the naked eye. When she awakened, she rushed to the den, took down the picture of Lincoln, and when she pressed the button revealed in the dream, an opening appeared containing the black box, which in turn contained a large sum in currency.

She discovered the treasures of her subconscious, which knows all, sees all, and has the know-how of accomplishment.

During a conversation with a successful businessman, he told me how he got the money to invest in a business partnership with another man. He had read *The Power of Your Subconscious Mind*, and one night he said to his subconscious prior to sleep, "You are all-wise. You know the answer to everything. I am interested in two gold stocks. Reveal to me which one I should buy for a quick profit." He relaxed, let go completely, and dropped off into a deep sleep. In a dream, a man appeared offering him a well-known product of one of the companies in which he was considering investing. He awakened and knew immediately that in the dream, his subconscious had offered him guidance regarding how to invest.

He bought several thousand shares of the stock of the company whose product had been in his dream, and in a short period of time it went up 40 points, netting him a tidy profit that enabled him to pay for a one-half interest in a thriving business.

Techniques for Harnessing the Power of Sleep and Dreams

I gave the following formula to a woman who said she had to take two sleeping tablets every night because she was so tense: In bed, talk to your body as follows: My toes are relaxed, my ankles are relaxed, my feet are relaxed, my legs are relaxed, my abdominal muscles are relaxed, my heart and lungs are relaxed, my spine is relaxed, my hands and arms are relaxed, my shoulders are relaxed, my neck is relaxed, my brain is relaxed, my eyes are relaxed, my facial muscles are relaxed. I now feel God's peace flowing through me, permeating my being. I sleep in peace; I wake in joy.

She quietly repeated these simple truths every night, knowing her body is subject to her thoughts. After a week or so of practicing this discipline, she has had no further trouble. She has discovered the meaning of these great truths.

You can discover the miracle-working power of your subconscious by plainly stating to your subconscious prior to sleep that you wish a certain specific thing accomplished. As you're dropping off to sleep, simply say either "Answer" or "Give your attention to this and reveal an answer to me." Do this either silently or audibly. You will be delighted to discover that forces within you will be released, leading to the desired result.

Charles Baudoin was a professor at the Rousseau Institute in France and a research director of the New Nancy School of Healing. He taught that the best way to impress the subconscious mind was to enter into a drowsy, sleepy state, or a state akin to sleep in which all effort was reduced to a minimum. Then in a quiet, passive, receptive way, by reflection, he would convey the idea to the subconscious. The following is his formula: "A very simple way of securing this (impregnation of the subconscious mind) is to condense the idea that is to be the object of suggestion, to sum it up in a brief phrase that can be readily graven on the memory, and to repeat it over and over again as a lullaby."

A good technique to practice prior to sleep is to cleanse your mind of all negatives and fill your mind with the truths of God, wishing love and goodwill to all. Affirm, "I sleep in peace, I wake in joy, and I live in God."

Your conscious mind controls your subconscious. You can use your conscious mind to alter the nature of your dreams, stopping the recurrence of "bad dreams," "nightmares," or dreams you dread, by employing the same techniques you use during the day to reject your negative thoughts. In this way, the habit of dream-control gradually will come under your own jurisdiction.

Often, "bad dreams" occur if you watch violent or horror dramas on television or read a murder/mystery or scary novel before going to sleep. If you find that you begin to have recurring "bad dreams" or nightmares and you suspect some activity that you are engaged in before going to bed is the source, affirm prior to sleep, "I know why I am dreaming this way, and I know it is a dream. I remain dreaming and the nightmare ceases and is switched off. God's love fills my soul, and I dream in peace all night and I wake in joy."

One of the best times for tapping the wisdom of your subconscious mind for ideas, answers, and inspiration is prior to sleep. The reason for this is that, generally speaking, you are more relaxed, at ease, and you are ready for quietude and deep sleep. Turn your request over to your subconscious, and then lull yourself to sleep with the phrase, "Answer me in a dream," or "Give your attention to this and reveal to me an answer in a dream." Knowing that your subconscious is responsive to you, do this with complete faith that you will receive the answer.

※

It is wise to have a pencil or tape recorder near you when you sleep, so that when you awaken you can jot down or recall the impressions that came to you in your dreams. You may be greatly surprised by what wisdom has been given to you in your sleeping state.

※

Some people say, "I never dream." We all dream. If you don't remember your dreams, suggest to your subconscious before you drop off to sleep two words: "I remember." It knows what you want to remember and will faithfully follow your instructions.

If you are aware of having had a dream but you cannot remember its contents, and you believe that it was important, you can also say those two words to yourself immediately upon awakening; as you practice this, the dream will come back in full form.

※

As you drift off to sleep, affirm: In a dream, Infinite Intelligence in my subconscious mind reveals to me the answer regarding _____ [your concern].

Principles to Remember and Apply

▶ In the sleepy state, you avoid conflict between your conscious and subconscious. Imagine the fulfillment of your desire over and over again prior to sleep. Then sleep in peace and wake in joy.

▸ If you have difficulty sleeping, talk to your body, telling it to relax and let go. Your body will obey you. Then affirm slowly and quietly, "I sleep in peace and I wake in joy, for He careth for me."

▸ When you go to sleep, your conscious concern is creatively joined to your subconscious mind, and the latter determines the way the answer or healing will take place.

▸ Dreams are dramatizations of your subconscious mind, usually appearing in symbolic form. Your disciplined imagination can unclothe the dream and reveal its hidden content.

▸ Prior to sleep, charge your subconscious with the task of evolving an answer to any problem, and prove its miracle-working power to yourself. It will answer you.

▸ Your subconscious speaks to you symbolically in dreams; however, you can suggest to your subconscious every night, "I dream literally and clearly." Your constant reiteration of that suggestion prior to sleep causes your subconscious to speak to you in literal terms.

▸ If you suffer from nightmares, you can change your nightmares by affirming before you go to sleep, "I remain dreaming and the nightmare ceases and is switched off. God's love fills my soul, and I dream in peace all night and I wake in joy."

▸ Dreams can symbolically warn you of impending danger or inform you of a future event for the good before either happens.

‣ Many times, as you think of the answer prior to sleep you will find that the entire formula or solution may appear in a dream. It is done unto you as you believe.

‣ The best time to tap the subconscious is prior to sleep, when you are relaxed, at peace, and ready for quietude and deep sleep.

Part II

ENRICH YOUR LIFE WITH THE UNLIMITED POWER OF YOUR SUBCONSCIOUS MIND

11 Your Unlimited Power to Overcome Worry and Fear

All the water in the ocean will not sink even
a small boat if the water doesn't get inside
the boat.
Likewise, all the problems, challenges, and
difficulties in the world cannot sink you, as long as
you do not permit them to get inside you.

Remember, thought is prayer. When you worry, you are actually praying for what you don't want. The subconscious mind takes your fears as a request and proceeds to bring them into your experience.

Don't try to run away from your worries and fears. Wherever you go, you take your mind with you—and the only place your worry or fear exists is in your mind.

Once, while traveling by train, I noticed a man carrying a bag on his back. The conductor said to him: "You can take that bag off your back. The train can carry both of you." There are a great many people carrying the burden of grief, sorrow, grudges, peeves, bitterness, and hostility on their backs, which robs them of vital energy, creating short circuits in their lives. *Cast thy burden upon the Lord (Law), and he shall sustain thee.* (Psalm 55:22)

When fear knocks at the door of your mind, or when worry, anxiety, and doubt cross your mind, remind yourself that your imagination took you to your worry. It can also take you to freedom and peace of mind.

Worry and fear cause pain; love and goodwill bring peace and health. *There is no fear in love; but perfect love casteth out fear: because fear hath torment. He that feareth is not made perfect in love.* (1 John 4:18)

Your worry is your mind's acceptance of negative conditions. It is having greater faith in your problem than in God and His Cosmic Wisdom. All fears and worries, therefore, are types of negative thinking. *Be strong and of good courage, be not afraid, neither be thou dismayed, for the Lord thy God is with thee whithersoever thou goest.* (Joshua 1:9)

Do not dwell on obstacles. Agree in your mind that what you desire is already present, that what you are seeking is seeking you, that the law of attraction will cause what you desire to come to you—and your worries will then flee.

When you say, "There is no way out. It's hopeless," then you live in the darkness and confusion created by your belief.

When next beset with worries or fears, ask yourself, "How am I using Cosmic Power?"

Know that the creator is greater than the creation. You have created your worries and fears, and you can equally rise above them. Remember, you have dominion over your thoughts, feelings, actions, and reactions in life. Live joyously and walk the earth with praise forever on your lips.

For verily I say unto you, That whosoever shall say unto this mountain, Be thou removed, and be thou cast into the sea; and shall not doubt in his heart, but shall believe that those things which he saith shall come to pass; he shall have whatsoever he saith. (Mark 11:23)

The truth of these words will never let you down but will supply you with infinite power for perfect living. The *mountain* stands for the difficulties, challenges, and problems confronting you. They may seem overwhelming, overpowering, and worrisome, but if you have faith in the Infinite Power within you and do not doubt it, you will affirm boldly, "Be thou removed," and your subconscious, hearing your bold and sincere decree, will begin withdrawing your worrisome thoughts from you.

※

Read the morning newspaper in any metropolitan area and you will find yourself caught up with worries: murder, crime, purse-snatching, rape, corruption in high places, and venality on the bench and in the legislative chambers. Remember, however, that all of these are of human origin, and you can *come out from among them and be separate.* (II Corinthians 6:17)

Align yourself with the principles of right action, harmony, love, joy, and beauty. All of these are attributes, qualities, and potencies of God, and they are within you. When you dwell on these qualities and contemplate the truths of God, you rise above the injustice and the cruelties of the world and you build a conviction counter to all its injurious beliefs and erroneous concepts.

You have a Divine immunity—a sort of spiritual antibody—to the occupations and preoccupations of the mass mind.

※

When fear or worry thoughts come to your mind, remind yourself that God is bringing your desire, ideal, plan, or purpose to pass in Divine Order. Affirm: "Infinite Intelligence gave me this desire, and it is now backing me up, revealing to me the perfect plan for its unfoldment, and I rest in that conviction." Continue in this attitude of mind until the day breaks and the shadows flee away.

※

You can decide to think whatever you choose about anything. What you have lost or suffered has nothing to do with the way you decide to think about it.

If you think of the Infinite Intelligence, or God, your thought neutralizes and destroys thoughts of fear, worry, lack and doubt, in the same manner as the sun dissolves the mist or the light casts out darkness.

*T*ake us the foxes, the little foxes, that spoil the vines: for our vines have tender grapes. (Song of Solomon 2:15)

Your problems are due to the "little foxes that spoil the vine": worry, fear, and negativity. These are the true "little foxes" that spoil the wine of life, which is the exhilarating and vitalizing flow of Infinite Supply coursing through your entire system.

You are the master of your thought reactions. You can order your thoughts around as you like, giving attention to whatever you choose to meditate on. You are a monarch in your conceptual realm. You can refuse a passport to any foreign visitors—such as fear, worry, negativity, anger, or hatred that try to enter your kingdom. You can order your subjects—thoughts and feelings—according to your desires, and they must obey you. You are the absolute monarch in your mental kingdom, with power to eliminate all enemies (worries, fears, negative thoughts) from your kingdom.

※

Worry and fear thoughts are not real; they deny that which is actual. Worry and fear are false beliefs of the mind. False beliefs will die if you refuse to give them attention.

※

Learn the great truth that no person, situation, or condition causes you to be unhappy or lonesome, or to suffer from pecuniary embarrassment. It is the beliefs and impressions made in your subconscious mind that cause these experiences in your life.

※

Worry of any kind is nature's alarm signal that you are believing wrongly. A change of thought will set you free.

※

Fear is a denial of the power of God and the goodness of God. Fear is faith upside down. Fear and worry are shadows in the mind; they are merely a conglomeration of sinister shadows, and shadows have no reality.

※

Is not that which you are afraid of merely a thought in your mind?

※

Every failure in life is a stepping-stone to your triumph.

Those who find God within themselves lose their self-doubt, worry, and fear.

All your fears, anxieties, and forebodings are caused by your belief in external powers and malevolent agencies. This is wrongful thinking. The only immaterial creative power is your thought, and once you are aware of the creative power of your thought and that thoughts are things, you are at once delivered from all bondage.

Cease transferring the power that is within you to things, conditions, people, or circumstances.

Henry Wadsworth Longfellow said, "Look not mournfully into the Past. It comes not back again. Wisely improve the Present. It is the thine. Go forth to meet the shadowy Future, without fear, and with a manly heart."

If you truly understand that there is only One Power and that in this Power there is only the principle of beauty, but none of ugliness; only the principle of harmony, but none of discord; only the principle of love, but none of hatred; only the principle of joy, but none of sadness; only the principle of opulence and abundance, but none of deprivation and poverty; and only the principle of right action, but none of wrong action, then you will know that fear and worry have no substance.

People who worry always expect things to go wrong. They will tell you all the reasons why something bad could happen, and not one reason why something good should or could happen. Such worry makes them weaker and less able to meet any challenges that might come along, as they attract exactly the conditions upon which they are mentally dwelling.

The fearful, worrisome perspective we impress upon our subconscious minds practically guarantees that some corresponding challenge or difficulty will erupt.

Whenever the idea comes to you that you must have something and it must appear on a certain day, remember that attitude of mind is one of tension, anxiety, and fear. You are already magnifying the ordinary attitude of mind of worry. Identify with Infinite Intelligence; then claim that Divine guidance will bring about what it is that you desire. Maintain that conviction and your contact with Infinite Intelligence within, and the day will break and your shadows will flee away.

Remember this important truth: One thing you can be absolutely certain about in this universe is that the laws of Infinite Intelligence within you of healing, guidance, and harmony are constant and invariable. Then arrange to live your life accepting this truth, and you will banish from your life forever all worries and fears.

▨

Worry comes from not making a habit of prayer and having no real contact with Infinite Power, from which you could draw strength and security.

▨

You believe you are cursed with your worries because of outside circumstances. In reality, however, worries are thoughts. You are the only thinker in your universe; you alone can overcome them. When you worry, you are using your mind negatively and destructively.

▨

When you are under mental stress or filled with fearful concerns and are carrying these around with you, the ordinary business of your life gets shortchanged.

▨

Do not spend time wrestling with your worries and fears. Do not *fight* a problem; *overcome* it.

▨

Fear thoughts, worry thoughts, or negative thoughts of any kind will not hurt you unless you entertain them for a long period of time and emotionalize them deeply. Otherwise, they will flow through you without doing the least damage. Potentially they may be trouble, but only if you allow them to become actualized. Your fears cannot be actualized unless you emotionalize them. At that stage, you begin to impress your subconscious mind with your worries and fears, and whatever is impressed in the subconscious mind will come to pass.

※

All conditions, circumstances, and events are subject to alteration. Every created thing will someday pass away. The age-old maxim, "This too shall pass away," is always true. The reality and realization of this can be a cause of fear and worry, unless you remind yourself that God is the same yesterday, today, and forever.

※

One of the main reasons for the feeling of insecurity, and thus for feelings of worry and fear, is that you are regarding the externals of life as causes, not realizing that they are really effects. Remember that the cause is within you, in your thoughts and feelings.

※

If you have not learned about your own essential greatness and the infinite riches within you, you will tend to magnify the problems and the difficulties that confront you. You will empower them, giving them the influence and control that you should rightly keep for yourself.

※

It is said that fear is our greatest enemy. This is true, because fear is behind failure.

⬚

Timidity is a state of mind that results from fear and worry. "Do the thing you are afraid to do," said Ralph Waldo Emerson, "and the death of fear is certain."

⬚

We are born with only two fears: the fear of falling and the fear of noise. These could be called our normal fears. They are a sort of alarm system given you by nature as a means of self-preservation. Normal fear is good. You hear an automobile coming down the road, for example, and you step aside to survive. The fear of being run over is overcome by your action. All other fears are abnormal fears, given to you by parents, relatives, teachers, and all those who influenced your early years.

Abnormal fears take over when we let our imaginations run riot.

Most of the things we fear do not exist; we bring them to pass by constantly fearing, believing, and expecting them. As Job said, *the thing which I greatly feared come upon me.* (Job 3:25)

⬚

A certain amount of anxiety is normal and necessary. It is excessive and prolonged tension that is dangerous. It's when you wind up the clock too tightly that you break the spring.

⬚

I am exceedingly joyful in all our tribulation.
(II Corinthians 7:4)

To be *joyful in all your tribulation* does not mean that you rejoice in having worries and fears, but rather that in the midst of them you can feel peace, knowing that there is an Infinite Healing Presence that is always willing to heal and restore you, provided you open your mind and heart to receive it.

If you are dwelling worrisomely over past actions or events, you are thinking of them *now*, the mental agony you are experiencing is in fact pain in your *present* moment. Likewise, if you are fearful about the future, you are in fact fearing it *now*, you are robbing and stealing joy, health, happiness, and peace of mind from your present moment.

The past and the future are two arch-thieves. Get rid of these two thieves. You have control over your present thoughts; direct them into the right channels.

Remember, there is no principle of hate, only of love. Love, therefore, is *now*. There is no principle of failure, only success. Success, therefore, is *now*.

Now is the time.

Now is the *only* time.

What thoughts are you thinking now?

And, behold, there arose a great tempest in the sea, insomuch that the ship was covered with the waves. . . . And his disciples came to him . . . saying, Lord, save us: we are perishing. (Matthew 8:24–25)

When you let yourself become beset with worries and fears, you are allowing yourself to be caught up in the tempest of worldly confusion, fear, and human opinion. You fear you will perish. But when you remember that Infinite Intelligence within you is All-Wise and All-Knowing, then you will be looking at the solution, the way out, the happy ending, ignoring the winds and the waves of worry and fear, and your ways will be ways of peace. *Then he arose, and rebuked the winds and the sea, and there was a great calm.* (Matthew 8:26)

HOW HE OVERCAME WORRY AND FEAR

During a world lecture tour, I had a two-hour conversation with a prominent government official. He had a deep sense of inner peace and serenity. He said that all the abuse he receives politically from newspapers and the opposition party never disturb him. His practice was to sit still for fifteen minutes in the morning and realize that in the center of himself was a deep, still ocean of peace. Meditating in this way, he generates tremendous power, which overcomes all manner of difficulties and fears.

He told me that at one time, a colleague called him at midnight and told him a group of people were plotting against him. This is what he said to his colleague, "I am going to sleep now in perfect peace. You can discuss the matter with me tomorrow morning at ten o'clock."

He said to me, "I know that no negative thought can ever manifest unless I emotionalize the thought and accept it mentally. I refuse to entertain their suggestion of fear. Therefore, no harm can come to me."

Techniques for Overcoming Worry and Fear

Follow these three steps to removing worries and fears.

First, take all your attention away from all thoughts of past and present hurts, grievances, resentments, fears, worries, sicknesses, defeats, discouragement, or lack of any kind.

Second, stop every negative thought by immediately substituting constructive thoughts, such as harmony, peace, love, joy, right action, and Divine guidance.

Third, take time out morning and evening to implant in your subconscious mind the mental patterns of harmony, abundance, security, success, serenity, and full expression.

When your mind is disturbed, a wonderful technique of healing is to become absorbed by nature, where beauty, order, symmetry, rhythm, and proportion prevail. When your mind is projected on the order and beauty of nature, your mind is transformed and renewed, which results in healing.

Your emotion follows thought. You can decide how you shall react to conditions, circumstances, and environment. If unpleasant news comes to you, if others criticize, condemn, and vilify you, remember that no one can hurt or injure you unless you give permission through your mental consent. Refuse permission. Do not allow any thought to disturb you. Positively refuse to react worrisomely or fearfully. Say, "I remain unmoved and undisturbed; nothing affects me except my own thought, and then only through my own mental consent."

When the impulse to worry comes, remind yourself that the law of thought is creative and that through the same process by which you have enlivened worries for yourself, you can create joy and happiness and confidence.

When I was about ten years old, I accidentally fell into a pool and went down three times. I can still remember the dark water engulfing my head, and my gasping for air until another boy pulled me out at the last moment. For years I feared the water.

An elderly psychologist said to me, "Go down to the swimming pool, look at the water, and say out loud in strong tones, 'I am going to master you. I can dominate you.' Then go into the water, take lessons, and overcome it." This I did, and I mastered the water.

Later, in my adult life, there was a time when I was filled with unutterable fear when standing before an audience. The way I overcame it was to stand before the audience, do the thing I was afraid to do, and the death of fear was certain.

Affirm positively that you, too, are now going to master your fears. Come to a definite decision in your conscious mind about this, and you will release the power of the subconscious, which will then flow in response to the nature of your thought.

The Greeks said that laughter is of the gods. Laughter is a medicine for many troubles. Laughter restores your perspective, takes your attention from yourself. Make it a special point to laugh at your fears, to laugh when people irritate you, and by all means to laugh at all the foolish, silly mistakes you made during the day. Laugh at yourself for being so stuffy and so serious. The greater the problem, the more humor you need. There can be no self-pity, and thus neither worry nor fear, when laughter takes over your soul.

When worrisome or fearful thoughts come to your mind, immediately affirm, "Infinite Intelligence is within me."

Here is an excellent thought to affirm in the midst of worry or fear: *The Lord is my shepherd, I shall not want; he leadeth me beside still waters; he restoreth my soul and leadeth me in the paths of righteousness. Yea, though I walk through the valley of the shadow of death, I will fear no evil. Surely goodness and mercy shall follow me all the days of my life. Of what should I be afraid?* (Psalm 23)

If God be for us, who can be against us? (Romans 8:31) Personalize this verse, and you will overcome all sense of self-doubt, worry, and fear: If God is *for me* who can be against me?

Principles to Remember and Apply

) Stand up to your worries and fears. Do the thing you are afraid to do, and the death of fear is certain.

) Fear and worry are destructive thoughts in your mind. Supplant them with constructive thoughts.

) Fear is behind all failure.

▶ You were born with only two fears: the fear of falling and the fear of noise. These are normal fears. All your other fears are abnormal. Get rid of them.

▶ If you think worrisome thoughts, worries follow; if you think good thoughts, good follows.

▶ Learn to laugh at your fears. That is the best medicine.

▶ If you really want to banish fear, you must give up your jealousies, hatreds, peeves, and grudges.

▶ Don't fight fear with fear. Meet it with the direct declaration, "Infinite Intelligence within me is the only Presence and Power; there is nothing to fear."

▶ A certain amount of tension is good; excess tension is destructive.

▶ There is always a solution to every problem. Contemplate the happy ending; what you contemplate, you experience.

▶ Affirm, "If God be *for me*, who can be against me?" and you will overcome all sense of self-doubt, worry, and fear.

▶ Worry is God's alarm, reminding you that you are thinking wrongly, and you should redirect your thinking processes immediately.

12 Your Unlimited Power to Overcome Negative Thinking

Don't place obstacles in your own way by thinking negatively.

▧

*T*o flourish and thrive, you need a special mental and spiritual diet. You are fed daily through the five senses by an avalanche of sights, sounds, and sundry concepts, both good and bad. Most of this food is highly unsavory. You must learn to turn inward to God and be replenished from the standpoint of Truth, rather than negativity.

Develop a healthy spiritual diet for your mind. Wonders will happen.

▧

The instant you receive the stimulus of a negative thought, supplant it with the mood of love and goodwill. If you fill your mind with love, negative thoughts cannot enter.

▧

Jealousy is a negative thought and a mental poison. It arises from a deep-seated fear or mistrust of another plus a feeling of guilt and uncertainty about oneself. Jealous people poison their own banquets and then eat them. The jealous person demands exclusive devotion and is intolerant of rivalry. The jealous person is suspiciously watchful.

"Oh, beware of jealousy;" wrote Shakespeare, "it is the green-eyed monster, which doth mock the meat it feeds on."

As Sunday night comes, many people talk about "blue Monday." These people are already resigning themselves to their "fate" and beginning to shut down their lives. Monday then comes with a certain sense of resignation: On Sunday they were consciously decreeing their future, and their subconscious responded accordingly. In all probability, they didn't even know that they had planned ahead and had thus created their "fate."

When you cohabit mentally with negative thoughts, your Life Force gets snarled up in your subconscious mind in the same way that when you put your foot on the garden hose, you block the flow of water. The negative emotions that are dammed up in your subconscious then come forth as all manner of diseases, both mental and physical.

Cast out negativism, ill will, criticism, and self-condemnation, and instead fill your mind with constructive thoughts of harmony, health, peace, joy, and goodwill, and you will be transforming your life.

▦

By thinking constructively, based on universal principles, you can change all the negative patterns in your mind and thereafter live a charmed life. Filling your mind with the truths of God, you neutralize, obliterate, and expunge from your mind everything unlike God—and you avoid all negative experiences.

▦

*L*et every man be swift to hear, slow to speak, slow to wrath. (James 1:19)

Be swift in hearing good news and never indulge in negative thinking or in the mood of anger. When such attitudes prevail, go within yourself at once and reclaim the feeling of being what you long to be.

▦

When you are loyal and devoted mentally to your ideal, the fear or the negative thought dies, and the ideal becomes real.

▦

The radio, television, and newspapers pour forth negative and despairing suggestions, but many people are not affected by them at all. You, too, have the power to reject all negative and destructive suggestions, because you are the only thinker in your universe, and you can choose your thoughts.

You become what you condemn. When you vilify, criticize, and find fault with others, you begin to exemplify what you criticize. Moreover, when you are angry, hostile, and bitter, your mind is much more receptive to the negative, fearful, and hateful suggestions of the world.

To walk the royal road to riches of all kinds—spiritual, mental, material, and financial—you must never place obstacles and impediments in the pathway of others; neither must you be jealous, envious, or resentful of others. Remember, your thoughts are creative and whatever you think about another you are creating in your own life and experience. Don't place obstacles in your own way by thinking negatively about another.

A negative thought or suggestion by another person has no power unless you give it power. Suggestions are *a* power, but they are not *the* Power (God) that moves as harmony, beauty, love, and peace. When those around you are expressing negativity or are casting negative suggestions toward you, always remember that you have the ability to unite mentally with the Infinite Intelligence within you, whose principles are love, generosity, and harmony— not negativity.

When a negative or angry thought comes to your mind, immediately supplant it with a spiritual thought, such as "The Peace of the universe fills my soul." As you do this regularly, all harmful thoughts will cease to come, and peace will come into your mind.

▩

Never finish a negative statement; reverse it immediately and wonders will happen in your life.

▩

If you have indulged in fear, worry, and other destructive forms of thinking, your subconscious mind will have accepted your negative thoughts as requests and will proceed to bring them into your experience. The remedy is to begin devoting your thoughts to kindness, peace, and forgiveness. Your subconscious mind, being creative, will then equally proceed to create the attributes in your life that you have earnestly decreed.

▩

Every time you think or say negative thoughts, you help prolong the situation that is wrecking your peace of mind. In effect, you are praying against yourself. Make your inner, silent thought conform to your desired aim.

▩

Thoughts generate emotions, and emotions kill or cure. To think negatively is to kill love, harmony, peace, beauty, and joy within you. Destructive emotions like negativity have a toxic effect not only on your mind and heart, but also on the very cells of your body.

Failure is negative thinking. It has many causes. One of them, perhaps the most crucial, is the conviction that failure is inevitable.

Your habitual thinking—what you regularly feel, believe, and give mental consent to, consciously or unconsciously—is imprinted on your subconscious mind. Every part of your being then expresses these thoughts.

How, and what, are you thinking today?

When you think negatively about others, the trouble is in your own thought-life. Other people are not responsible for the way you think about them. There is no one to change but yourself.

The cause of any unwanted, negative habit is negative and destructive thinking. The cure is to think of your freedom from the habit and to feel the thrill of accomplishment.

Your subconscious mind has tremendous power. Influence it only positively, constructively, and harmoniously, because it will not argue controversially. Whatever orders (thoughts) you give it will be obeyed. You do great injury to yourself, therefore, by the negative thoughts you entertain, as your subconscious will accept your negative thoughts as your wishes.

Every part of your being then expresses these thoughts; your outer life will demonstrate what you are consciously impressing in your subconscious mind. Never affirm inwardly, therefore, anything you do not want to experience outwardly.

You may be deceived by error, but the Truth remains forever undimmed by time. Align your thoughts and actions with the principles of the Infinite Intelligence within you, and you will neutralize all the harmful effects of the negatives implanted in your subconscious mind.

HOW THEY TRANSFORMED THEIR NEGATIVE THINKING

One day a man from San Francisco flew down to see me. He was extremely tense. His doctor had diagnosed his condition as anxiety neurosis. He was very successful financially and was sales manager of a very big corporation. The president and vice president of the corporation liked him and respected him.

As we talked, the real cause of his trouble came to light. A classmate of his was sales manager of a rival corporation but had been promoted to the position of president of the corporation. This man admitted that he was envious of his classmate's promotion. He was mentally competing with him. He said, "You know, that guy beat me at everything in school and college; he even took away the girl I loved and married her."

I explained to him that the only true competition there was in life was that which existed between the idea of success and the idea of failure in his own mind, and that he was born to win, not fail; for the Infinite could not fail. Therefore, all he had to do was to focus his attention on success and then all the powers of his subconscious would back him up and compel him to succeed, as the law of the subconscious is compulsive.

He began to see that the past is dead and that nothing matters but this moment. As he changed his present thoughts and kept them changed, his whole world would magically melt into the image and likeness of his contemplation.

I also explained to him that by entertaining envious thoughts he was actually impoverishing himself, and that this was one of the worst possible attitudes to hold, because his negative thinking and his feelings of inferiority and envy and jealousy were playing havoc with his mental and emotional life, and would tend to block his expansion along all lines.

The remedy was very simple. I told him to bless and sincerely wish greater prosperity and success for his former classmate. After a few weeks, he discovered that the envious thoughts lost all power over him.

I once had an interesting chat with a young man named Cyril, who was studying mental discipline in Paris. We were both crossing the English Channel from Dover to Calais.

Cyril explained that from time to time he would examine his thoughts, and if he found himself holding angry, negative thoughts he would say to himself, "This is not the Infinite thinking, speaking, and acting in me. These are not of God; they are destructive and false. I now think, speak, and act from the standpoint of God and His love."

Every time Cyril was tempted to become angry, critical, depressed, or irritable, he would think of God and His love and peace, and the temptation would pass. This is internal discipline and spiritual understanding.

At the conclusion of my visit with a friend who was in the hospital, he urged me to talk to the man in the next bed, Robert C.

I introduced myself to Robert. He seemed glad to have a distraction. As we talked about the hospital, he suddenly said, "The worst part of being here is that I know Harry is gloating like anything. I loathe that man. They don't come any lower than him."

"Who's Harry?" I asked.

"He was my partner," Robert told me. "Then I found out he was cooking the books and diverting the company's assets. I barely managed to avoid bankruptcy as a result."

It was easy to see that Robert's loathing had become a festering psychic wound.

"Would you invite your former partner to dinner?" I asked.

"Only if I knew I could get away with poisoning him!" he declared.

"Yet you entertain him constantly in your mind," I pointed out, "and it is not he who is being poisoned. It is you. You give him—or rather, your psychic image of him—immense power over your mind, your body, and your vital organs. You are the only thinker in your universe. That means you are directly responsible for the thoughts, concepts, and images that come to you. If you saturate your mind with hatred and loathing, the effects will surely make themselves known in your body. But if you saturate your mind with the truths of God, only wholeness and health can follow."

A Technique for Overcoming Negative Thinking

The ideal way to rid yourself of unwanted emotions is to practice the law of substitution. Through the law of mental substitution, you substitute a positive, constructive thought for the negative thought. When negative thoughts enter your mind, do not fight them; instead, just say to yourself: "My faith is in all things good." You will find the negative thoughts disappear just as light dispels the darkness.

At times you will find your mind falling back into its old habits of fretting, fussing, worrying, and recounting the verdicts of others. When these thoughts come to your mind, issue the order, "Stop! My thoughts are the way I feed my subconscious." Do this a hundred times a day, or a thousand times, if necessary.

Principles to Remember and Apply

▶ When negativity knocks at the door of your mind, let faith in God and all things good open the door.

▶ Negativity is a mental poison. Forgiveness and love are the spiritual antidotes to use; then a healing follows.

▶ You can mentally transform all negative impressions that come to you through your five senses by using the law of substitution. Immediately substitute a positive, constructive thought for a negative one. The positive emotion will neutralize and destroy all negative emotions.

▶ You can protect yourself against any negative onslaughts from without by realizing and affirming: "God and I are one, and if God be for me, no one can be against me."

▶ *Never* finish a negative statement. After a while, the negative thoughts will cease to come, and you will have conditioned your subconscious to kindness, cooperation, and harmony.

▶ Never engage in such negative thinking as lack, limitation, loneliness, and frustration. *For as he thinketh in his heart, so is he.* (Proverbs 23:7)

▶ The negative thoughts of others have no power to reach you if you refuse to accept them, and they will return to their point of origin with double force.

▶ You can change any negative pattern of thought or action by reminding yourself that instead of fear, the Presence and Power that created the world in harmony is within you.

13 Your Unlimited Power to Achieve Prosperity

Realize that the whole world is yours to enjoy, and you will know how truly rich you already are, and you will know the key to prosperity.

▨

Wealth means possessing all the food, clothing, energy, vitality, health, happiness, inspiration, and creative ideas you desire.

▨

Realize that your thought is creative; that what you feel, you attract; that what you imagine, you become; that whatever you impress on your subconscious mind will be projected on the screen of space as form, function, experience, and events. If you talk about not having enough to go around, and about how little you have and how you must cut corners, those thoughts are only impoverishing you. Making such statements as "There isn't enough to go around," "I'll lose the house because of the mortgage," and so forth while seeking prosperity is like writing a check to yourself that will come back to you marked "Insufficient funds." In order to become rich and to solve your financial problems, you must continuously dwell on thoughts of wealth, prosperity, and success.

The secret of prosperity is to substitute the thoughts of lack and limitation with the habitual thoughts of the infinite and inexhaustible supply of God's riches. Change your thoughts and *keep them changed*. As you steer and direct your thoughts to the riches of the Infinite flowing into your experience, a fantastic difference will take place in your life.

The way to success and prosperity is already within you. You do not have to beg, supplicate, or beseech God. All you have to do is change the stream of your mental thought and imagery.

Do not ask for just enough to get by. You don't want just enough to get by. Be bold enough to claim that it is your right to be rich, and your deeper mind will honor your claim. You are here to lead the life more abundant.

Many people think that wealth, happiness, and abundance are not going to be theirs in this life, that these attainments are only for other people.

It is a Law that . . . *it is done unto you as you believe*. If *you* don't believe that you have the right to your heart's desire—be it prosperity or whatever—knowing that the law is impersonal, always responding to your belief, then it will not be a condition of life but your belief that will become your self-fulfilling prophecy.

⬚

Remember, any object to which you give special attention will tend to grow and magnify itself in your life. Attention is the key to life. Think of increase along all lines. Feel that you are successful and prosperous, since the feeling of wealth produces wealth.

⬚

Be sure you wish for all those around you success, happiness, and abundance, knowing that as you wish increase of wealth and happiness for others, they will pick up your thoughts subconsciously and will be benefited by the feeling of riches and abundance emanating from you. As you radiate abundance and riches to others, you are also attracting more of God's riches to yourself.

⬚

In talking with many people, I find that often the reason they do not prosper is that they think it is wrong to pray for wealth and success. Nothing could be further from truth. *I am come that they might have life, and that they have it more abundantly.* (John 10:10) Those who hesitate to claim prosperity and the good things of life deprive themselves of these available and visible blessings. You are here to lead the life more abundant, and unless you express abundance and prosperity and claim the riches of the Infinite, you may find yourself besieged by creditors and your family in need.

It is your God-given right to be rich. The law of life is abundance, not poverty.

⬚

This is a mental and spiritual universe. The world is Spirit, God, or Infinite Intelligence in form. Spirit and matter are one. Money may rightly be looked upon as the visible manifestation of Invisible abundance.

▨

Envy of the prosperity of others blocks the flow of your good. Envy of others exalts them and demotes you. God is your source of abundance, and your every want can be met instantly and perfectly. To be envious of others is to deny your own good and impoverish yourself. Envy is a waste of energy and is destructive to your prosperity. Moreover, the quickest way to cause wealth to take wings and fly away is to criticize and condemn others who have more wealth than you.

If you see someone depositing large sums of money in the bank or making a large purchase, and you have only a meager amount to deposit and are only able to make small purchases, does it make you envious? The way to overcome this is to say to yourself, "Isn't it wonderful! I rejoice in that person's prosperity. I wish for that person greater and greater wealth."

Bless those whose prosperity, success, and vast riches arouse your envy. By so doing you will heal your own state of mind and enter into the consciousness of one who, possessing all things, pours out of his or her inner and outer riches abundant gifts upon others. That is true prosperity.

▨

It is a great folly to not realize that the true riches are within yourself—in the Creative Power of your own mind—and to look, instead, upon external conditions as the source of true riches.

Do not give your allegiance, loyalty, and trust to created

things, but to the Creator, the Eternal Source of everything in the universe. Convince yourself in your mind that money is forever flowing freely in your life and that there is always a wonderful surplus. Then, should there be a financial collapse of banks, the stock market, employment, or the government tomorrow, you will be applying the laws of your subconscious in the right way and you will still attract wealth and be cared for. You will have all the money you want—*along with* peace of mind, harmony, wholeness, and serenity.

Remember that the channels through which you receive your wealth are not the source, and you should not confuse the two.

All transactions take place in the mind, and unless things are paid for and accepted mentally, one does not experience any result on the objective plane of life. The price you pay is belief. *According to your faith, be it unto you.* (Matthew 9:29) You must believe that you have the right to prosperity.

Your inner speech is the cause of all the outer experiences in your life. Think, speak, and act if you already had the money you are seeking. *For as he thinketh in his heart, so is he.* (Proverbs 23:7)

Some people think it is spiritually correct to avoid using the word "money" in their conversation; they speak of "supply," "abundance," and "prosperity," although what they really mean is money. They have old concepts and think it is wrong to desire money. This makes no sense and is very unreasonable.

Remember that your habitual thinking forms definite paths and tracks in your subconscious mind. You will always have plenty if you use the law of your mind in the right way and direct your inner speech correctly.

Wealth is the result of optimism and success habit-thinking, and poverty is the result of pessimism and failure habit thinking.

Money means freedom from want.

Don't affirm "There is no future for me, my salary is too small; I'll never get ahead." Likewise, don't repeatedly say, "I can't afford it." Your inner speech will be accepted by your subconscious mind and you will remain in that restricted and unhappy situation. Your subconscious mind takes your fear and negative statement as your request and proceeds in its own way to bring obstacles, delays, lack, and limitation into your life. It takes you at your word, seeing to it that you will not be in a position to do or purchase what you want.

Gaze on the lavishness, extravagance, and bounty of nature, and realize that there is an abundance of all things in this world. There is no shortage of God's wisdom or creative ideas. Humans, in their greed and lust, create an artificial shortage.

Walk in the consciousness of God's eternal supply. As long as you maintain this prosperity consciousness, you cannot suffer losses. No matter what form wealth takes, you will always be amply supplied.

Use the money you now have freely. Release it with joy, and realize that God's wealth flows to you in avalanches of abundance.

Infinite Intelligence within your subconscious can only do *for* you what it can do *through* you. Use your subconscious mind correctly, and wealth will flow to you in abundance.

Many people who come to me for advice regarding financial lack and insecurity make the following statement in common: "There is nothing wrong with me that $50,000 will not take care of."

I ask each one, "Do you believe in wealth?" Invariably they say, "Yes, of course, I see evidence of it everywhere," or words to that effect.

I then go on. "If you look around you as you walk down the street, you see temples, churches, banks, and stores equipped with all manner of merchandise; you see millions of automobiles and trucks and countless machines, all of which came out of the mind of some person. Every device, construction, and invention—such as radio, TV, automobile, computers, homes, skyscrapers—was once invisible; but someone had an idea or a thought-image in his or her mind, and nourishing the idea mentally and emotionally, that person's subconscious mind compelled him or her into action.

Moreover, that person then attracted everything necessary for the realization of his or her dreams. There is enough material in the world to clothe every man like a king and every woman like a queen. Nature is lavish, extravagant, bountiful, and wasteful. Look at the untold treasures in the earth and sea that have not yet been tapped."

After this preliminary discussion on the subject of wealth, my listeners begin to perceive that wealth is of the mind—just an idea or a thought-image—and that when this idea is energized and vitalized, the subconscious will activate the conscious mind, and the law of attraction will attract riches to them—spiritual, mental, and material.

░

If you are having financial difficulties, if you are trying to make ends meet, it means you have not convinced your subconscious mind that you will always have plenty—and some to spare.

░

Do not believe the story that the only way you can become wealthy is by the sweat of your brow and hard labor. It is not so; the effortless way of life is the best. Do the thing you love to do, and do it for the joy and thrill of it.

░

Perhaps you are like many who, when they said, "I am prosperous, I am wealthy," they felt within that they were lying to themselves. One man told me, "I have affirmed that I am prosperous until I am tired. Things are now worse. I knew when I made the statement that it was obviously not true." His affirmations were being continually rejected by the conscious mind, and the very opposite of what he outwardly affirmed and claimed was made manifest. You will not get results if ten minutes after you make your affirmations of prosperity, you indulge in fear thoughts or self-doubt, neutralizing the good you had affirmed.

※

Entertaining negative, envious, lack-and-limitation thoughts places you in a very negative position. Remember: Wealth flows *from* you, not *to* you.

※

If you are critical about someone whom you claim is making money dishonestly, cease giving thought to that person. That person is using the law of mind negatively; the law of mind will take care of that person.

Remember: The block or obstacle to your wealth is in *your own* mind, not someone else's mind or actions. Get on good terms with your own mind.

※

I once talked with a minister who had a very good following. He had excellent knowledge of the laws of mind and was able to impart this knowledge to others—but he could never make ends meet! He had what he thought was a good alibi for his plight, by quoting from Timothy: For *the love of money is the root of all evil.* (I Timothy 6:10) He neglected what followed in the seventeenth verse of the same chapter, when Paul charges the people to place their trust or faith in the living God, *who giveth us richly all things to enjoy.* (I Timothy 6:17)

The Bible does not say that *money* is the root of all evil, it says that *the love of money* is the root of all evil. Love of money to the exclusion of everything else will cause you to become lopsided and unbalanced.

If you were physically ill, you would not consider that condition to be your unalterable destiny. Instead, you would think, "There is something wrong with me," and you would do something about the condition at once.

Think of yourself in the same way if you are suffering from prosperity illness.

Make service to others your primary goal, and your prosperity is assured.

Getting rich or advancing in life is not a matter of being in a certain business or a certain location or having a certain talent. Some people of great talent remain poverty-stricken and frustrated, while others who have very little talent or education prosper beyond their fondest dreams. Riches are of the mind.

When the Infinite Thinker thought of a sequoia tree, He did not cause the instant formation of a full-grown tree, He just started in motion all the forces necessary to produce the tree through the subjective wisdom operating in the seed.

Likewise, when you desire to be free from all financial problems, you must realize that you, too, are a thinker, that your thoughts, too, are creative, and that you can originate ideas, images, plans, and purposes. That does not mean, however, that when you open your eyes, all the wealth necessary to immediately alter your circumstances will necessarily be lying before you. What it means is that you cannot create anything in this world until you have *thought* that something into existence.

Then, believe and accept that success is your Divine right and that Life will reward you—and as you believe, it shall be done unto you.

Someone once brought to my attention a statement by Henry Ford. When he was asked what he would do if he lost all his money and his business, he replied, "I would think of some other fundamental, basic need of all people, and I would supply that need more cheaply and more efficiently than anyone else. In five years I would again be a multimillionaire."

Wealth and poverty have their origins in your own mind. Like Henry Ford, you must come to a clear-cut decision that you intend to be wealthy and successful.

Do you have a poverty complex?

Many persons have the idea or dominant thought that they must chase after wealth, else they will lose it.

When anxious thoughts about debts come to mind, never think of bills or lack or debts, but smilingly give thanks for God's abundance and riches, and rejoice that the obligation is paid now. When you do this, there is a reconditioning of the mind to wealth.

※

A person who is poor—that is, a person who doesn't know how to operate and release the riches of his or her mind—can at any time he or she wishes begin to practice the law of opulence and again attract wealth, success, and riches of all kinds.

※

Cease looking down your nose, therefore, at material things. Every physical thing created is the Living Spirit within someone, manifesting as material form. If you are condemning anything in this world, you are demoting and depreciating yourself.

HOW THEY ACCEPTED PROSPERITY

I once had the most amazing telephone call from the husband of a woman whom I shall call Mrs. H, saying: "My wife just inherited a million dollars. You told her what to do."

Naturally, I congratulated him and wished for both of them all the blessings of life. I recalled talking to her one Sunday after a lecture in Los Angeles, at which time she had said that she wanted a million dollars for a certain project that was very sound and constructive. I explained to her that she first had to establish the mental equivalent of a million dollars in her mind, and that she could do this by getting intensely interested in the finished project, looking at it in her mind, rejoicing in the accomplished fact, and giving thanks for the wonder of it all.

She pictured the end in her mind, made it very vivid and real, and every night prior to sleep, she would affirm "a million, a million, a million," over and over again as a lullaby until she fell asleep, knowing her subconscious must sooner or later accept it. At the end of about a month, she was advised by an attorney that she had inherited over a million dollars. It was, as her husband said, "completely out of the blue."

There was a young lady who regularly came to my lectures and classes. She had to change buses three times; it took her one and a half hours each time to come to the lectures. In one lecture I explained how a young man who needed a car in his work received one. She went home and experimented as outlined in my lecture. Here is her letter in part, narrating her application of my method, and published by her permission:

Dear Dr. Murphy:

This is how I received a Cadillac.

I wanted one to come to the lectures regularly. In my imagination I went through the identical process I would go through if I were actually driving a car. I went to the showroom, and the salesman took me for a ride in one. I also drove it several blocks. I claimed the Cadillac as my own over and over again.

I kept the mental picture of getting into the car, driving it, feeling the upholstery, etc., consistently for over two weeks. Last week I drove to your lectures in a Cadillac. My uncle in Inglewood passed away, and left me his Cadillac and his entire estate.

A salesman who attended my Sunday lectures and who listened to my daily radio program asked me, "How can *I* make $75,000 a year? I am married and have three children. I barely make ends meet. My wife has to work in order for us to break even!"

I explained to him that the thought-image or mental pattern in his mind is the *first cause* relative to the thing desired; it is the actual substance of the thing desired, untouched by any previous conditions of lack, limitation, or restrictions of any kind.

He concluded that all he had to do was to communicate his thought-image to his subconscious mind, and the result or manifestation of his idea would come forth.

The following is his letter to me, which followed our conversation.

Dear Dr. Murphy:

Every morning for the three months after I talked to you, I gave myself the mirror treatment. I stood before my mirror after shaving and decreed out loud, slowly, feelingly, and knowingly: "John, you are a tremendous success. You are making $75,000 a year. You are an outstanding salesman." I kept repeating this for about ten or twelve minutes every morning, knowing that finally I would build in my subconscious mind the mental equivalent of $75,000 and that I would succeed in psychologically impregnating myself with that amount. I was guided to take up public speaking; I gave a talk about ten weeks ago at our annual sales meeting. The vice president congratulated me, I was promoted, and I was given a more lucrative district. My commissions and salary in the past year have exceeded $75,000! Truly, the mind is the source of wealth and all the riches of Heaven.

I once had a most interesting conversation with a surgeon when I was in Killarney, Ireland. He and his charming wife were touring the country. We began to talk about the wonders of the mind, and he told me a fabulous story about his father. This is the essence of it, and I am going to present it in the simplest possible way.

This young surgeon was the son of a miner in Wales. His father had worked long hours at very low wages; as a boy, the surgeon had had to go to school barefoot as his father could not afford to buy shoes for him. Fruit and meat appeared on the table twice a year, mainly at Easter and at Christmas; buttermilk, potatoes, and tea represented the main diet of this family.

One day, this young man said to his father, "Dad, I want to be a surgeon, and I'll tell you why. The boy I am going to school with had cataracts; the eye surgeon operated on him, and now he sees perfectly. I want to do good like that doctor."

His father replied, "Son, I have set aside 3,000 pounds (about $8,000 at the time) which I have saved over a period of twenty-five years. It is set aside for you, but I would rather you not touch it until such time as you have finished your medical education. You then can use it to open up a beautiful office with all the accoutrements of your profession. In the meantime, the money will be drawing interest, and you will have security. You know that any time you really need it during your medical studies, you can always draw upon it. It is all yours, but I would prefer that you let it accumulate interest, and on your graduation it will be a nice nest egg for you."

This thrilled the young man beyond words, and he vowed never to touch the money until he graduated from medical school. He worked his way through medical school, working in pharmacies at night and during holidays; he also earned money as an instructor in pharmacology and chemistry in the medical college. His whole idea was to live up to his promise to his father that he would not touch the money in the bank until he graduated.

The day came when he graduated, and his father told him, "Son, I have been digging for coal all my life and have gotten nowhere. There is not a shilling or a penny in the bank and there never was. I wanted you to dig deeply and find the treasures in the gold mine within yourself, which is limitless, inexhaustible, and eternal."

"For a moment," the surgeon said, "I was flabbergasted, dumbfounded, and inarticulate. After a few minutes, I got over the consternation and the shock, and then both of us burst out laughing. Then I realized that what Dad had really wanted to teach me was the feeling of wealth engendered by the thought of plenty of money in the bank to back me up if I needed it. It gave me courage, faith, and confidence and made me believe in myself. My belief that I had 3,000 pounds in the bank had accomplished the purpose just as well as if it actually had been deposited in the bank in my name."

This surgeon remarked that all that he had accomplished externally was but a symbol of his inner faith, vision, and conviction. For every person in the world, the secret of success, accomplishment, achievement, and fulfillment of goals in life lies in the discovery of the miraculous power of his or her thought and feeling. Our surgeon friend acted confidently, just as if the money was always there!

A young lady, a very good writer who had had several articles accepted for publication, said to me, "I don't write for money." I said to her, "It's true that you don't write for money, but what's wrong with money? The laborer is worthy of his hire. What you write inspires, lifts up, and encourages others. When you adopt the right attitude, financial compensation will automatically come to you freely and copiously."

She actually disliked money. *She had a subconscious thought pattern that there was some virtue in poverty.* I explained to her that there was no evil in the universe and that good and evil were in the thoughts and motivations of people. All evil comes from mis-interpretation of life and misuse of the laws of mind. In other words, the only evil is ignorance, and the only consequence is suffering.

She began to practice this simple prayer, which multiplied money in her experience:

> My writings go forth to bless, heal, inspire, elevate, and dignify the minds and hearts of men and women, and I am Divinely compensated in a wonderful way. I look upon money as Divine substance, for everything is made from the One Spirit. I know matter and spirit are one. Money is constantly circulating in my life, and I use it wisely and constructively. Money flows to me freely, joyously, and endlessly. Money is an idea in the mind of God, and it is good and very good.

She completely eradicated the superstitious belief that money was evil, and her income tripled in three months.

Techniques for Attracting Prosperity

Silently give to all people you meet the following blessing: God gave you richly all things to enjoy, and you are prospered beyond your fondest dreams.

Affirm daily: There's plenty of money in the world, there's plenty of everything, and I know there are endless resources in my subconscious mind that I have never tapped.

Here is the master program for disciplining your mind for prosperity. If you follow this technique, you will never want for money all the days of your life.

Step 1: Realize that everything you see—the stars in the sky or the riches of the earth—came out of the invisible mind of God, or Life, and that everything any person invented or created came out of the invisible mind of that person, and that anything anyone has ever made came out of the mind of some person. Affirm that thoughts are things and that thoughts are creative.

Step 2: Acknowledge that as there is only one Mind, and that your mind and the mind of God are one, for there is only one Mind common to all, and that God (Mind) is the Source of your supply as He is the Source of the sun and the air you breathe, that it is as easy for God to create wealth in your life as it is for God to create a blade of grass.

Step 3: Engrave in your subconscious mind the idea of wealth, knowing that ideas are conveyed to the subconscious by repetition, faith, and expectancy. When you repeat a thought pattern or an act over and over again, it becomes automatic, and your subconscious, being compulsive, will be compelled to express it. It is the same as learning to walk, swim, play the piano, or type.

Step 4: Understand that you must *believe* in what you are affirming. Realize that what you are affirming is like the apple seeds you deposit in the ground: They grow after their kind. By watering and fertilizing those seeds, you accelerate their growth. If thoughts of lack or doubt come to you, such as, "I can't afford that trip" or "I can't pay that bill," never finish those negative statements. Reverse them immediately in your mind by affirming, "God is my instant and everlasting supply, and that bill is paid in Divine Order." If your desire is a new car, don't say, "I can't buy that." Say to yourself, "That car is for sale. It is a Divine idea, and I accept it in Divine Order." If negative thoughts come to you fifty times in one hour, reverse them each time by thinking, "God is my instant supply, meeting that need right now," or words to that effect. After a while, the thought of lack and disbelief will lose all momentum, and you will find your subconscious is being conditioned to wealth.

Step 5: Lull yourself to sleep every night by reiterating this great truth: "I am ever grateful for God's riches that are ever active, ever present, unchanging, and eternal."

Whenever you receive a bill in the mail, immediately give thanks that you have received that same amount. I have taught this magic formula to many, and in every case they have become eternally grateful for its benefits.

If you are concerned that you will not use money constructively and judiciously, quietly say throughout the day and before going to sleep, "Infinite Intelligence governs and watches over all my financial transactions." Do this frequently, and you will find that your money-use will be wise.

You may be in debt and have no funds, influence, or tangible assets; but if you begin to habitually and sincerely claim, "God's wealth is circulating in my life, and there always is a Divine surplus," wonders will soon happen in your life!

Principles to Remember and Apply

▶ Wealth is a thought-image in the mind, a state of mind. Believe in the law of riches, and you shall receive.

▶ Life itself is a gift to you; you are here to lead the abundant life, a life of happiness, joy, health, and rich living. Believe and expect the riches of the Infinite, and invariably the best will come to you.

▶ Infinite Intelligence in your subconscious can only do *for* you what it can do *through* you. Your thoughts and feelings control your attainment of riches.

▶ Be careful that when you affirm wealth, success, right action, and promotion, you do not subsequently deny what you affirm. Stop neutralizing your good.

▶ If you are envious or critical of those who have amassed wealth and honors, you will impoverish yourself along all lines. Wish for everyone what you wish for yourself. That is the key to your abundance.

▶ Bless others richly. Pour out the blessing of the Infinite on all those you envy, and you will open the door to countless blessings for yourself.

▶ Contemplate the abundance of nature and you will experience the life more abundant.

▶ The law of life is plenty, not lack.

▶ Make service to others your primary goal; then your prosperity is assured.

▶ Never use phrases like "I can't afford it" or "I can't do this." Remember, your subconscious mind does not argue with you. It accepts what your conscious mind decrees.

▶ Your dominant idea should be *wealth*, not *poverty*. Remember, if you criticize money or don't believe you will ever make enough, you will find yourself in want financially.

▶ If you're seeking prosperity but have no idea how to go about it, your subconscious will give you the idea you seek.

▶ Do not ask for just enough to get by. Claim that it is your right to be rich and your deeper mind will honor your claim.

▶ Give thanks that when you receive a bill, you have also received the money to pay it. The idea will gradually impregnate your subconscious mind.

▶ The idea of competition limits your supply. The riches of the universe are infinite.

▶ When faced with the problem of needing a certain amount of money on a certain date, forget the amount and the date, as this mental attitude tends to produce anxiety. Affirm, instead, that God is your instant and everlasting supply, meeting all your needs now and forevermore.

▶ Never procrastinate the realization of your good. Never say to yourself, "I must wait years for a promotion or an increase in salary." Your subconscious takes you literally, and when you say, "I'll have to wait," you are blocking your own good.

> ❯ The minute you admit there is such a thing as wealth, which you can see everywhere in nature's abundance, you will have no problem living in the joyous expectancy of God's riches— spiritual, mental, and material.

14 Your Unlimited Power to Attain Success

There is no success without peace of mind.

※

*T*he only chance you have is the one you make for yourself.

※

By blessing those whose promotion, success, and wealth annoy us or incite our envy or jealousy, and by wishing that they become even more prosperous and more successful in every way, you heal your own mind and open the door to the riches of the Infinite.

※

If you have the desire to make a better razor blade, better computer chips, a better snow shovel, or anything else, and your desire is to contribute to humanity in a constructive way and to practice the Golden Rule in all transactions, then you are about God's business, and God, by His very nature, will be for you. Then there is no power in heaven or on earth that can withhold from you success and prosperity.

▓

Serving people wisely and kindly is success and Divine love in action.

▓

God is always successful, whether making a star, a planet, a tree, or the cosmos—and what is true of God is true of you, for God dwells in you. Therefore, you were born to succeed, as the Infinite cannot fail. Acknowledge this in your mind and heart, and you will know that you *cannot* fail!

▓

Many people believe that their success is in God's hands, that they should accept what comes to them. This isn't the truth. The truth is that you are to take the initiative. God, or the Cosmic Power, does not work *for* you, but *through* you—through your thought and imagination.

▓

The way to success and prosperity is already within you. You do not have to beg, supplicate, or beseech God. All you have to do is change the stream of your mental thought and imagery.

▓

All successful men and women possess one outstanding characteristic, and that is their ability to make *prompt* decisions and to *persist* in carrying those decisions through to *completion*.

A distinguished businessman once told me that in his fifty years of experience in dealing with men and women in the commercial and industrial fields, he found that all those who failed had one characteristic in common: They hesitated to make decisions; they vacillated and wavered. Further, when they did make decisions, they were not persistent in adhering to them.

To be jealous of another's talents, success, achievements, or wealth is to demote yourself and attract to yourself lack, loss, and limitation. Actually, you are rejecting the Divine Source of all good and saying to yourself, "He or she can have those things and be successful, but I can't." This deprives you of success.

It is your inner thought, feeling, and imagery—in other words, your mental attitude—operating within you, rather than the winds and the waves of circumstances, that makes the difference between promotion and success, failure and loss. What you are experiencing is the exact reproduction of your habitual thinking and imagery.

To attain success, become a self-starter. Some people only "come to life" in emergencies, instead of making it a daily habit to abide continually in the field of potential energy.

※

Lord Chesterfield said: "Some men live and die with all their greatness still within them."

Failure to reach your goal or to attain your objective is to sin. The word *sin* is from a Greek word meaning to miss the mark. When the Greek archers failed to hit the bull's eye, it was said that they had sinned, or had missed the mark. Your goal, desire, objective, or ideal is the mark for which you are aiming. When you fail to express health, wealth, peace of mind, and true expression, you are sinning against Infinite Intelligence within you, which is ever ready to guide you and show you the way.

※

Your potential must be increased through your belief, commitment, and dynamic action, or it will move away from you.

※

When you want something, do not think of all the reasons why you can't have it, but realize there is an Infinite Intelligence that will attract to you what you want. As you accept this truth, the deeper currents of your mind will bring it to pass and you will achieve success.

※

A burning desire to be and to do is a prerequisite for accomplishment. Identify yourself with your goal; mentally and emotionally unite with it. As you do this, Infinite Intelligence will activate the power of your subconscious mind and bring your desired attainment to pass.

To mentally unite with the *idea* of success, and to know that you are thereby invoking a subjective power that responds to your habitual thinking, is to create success.

You possess all things by right of consciousness.

Two people who understood the secrets of success were Albert Einstein and Thomas Edison.

Einstein loved mathematics, and it revealed its secrets to him. He was engrossed and fascinated with the universe and its laws. He gave his attention, devotion, and industry to the subject of time, space, and the fourth dimension, and his subconscious responded by revealing the secrets of these subjects to him.

Edison experimented with, meditated on, and explained the principle of electricity. He had an intense desire to light up the world and serve mankind, and electricity yielded its secrets to him. He paid the price in perseverance, stick-to-itiveness, and confidence, knowing that the answer would come. He brought forth countless inventions because he paid the price first by giving attention, interest, and complete dedication to his project, knowing in his heart and soul that there was a subjective intelligence that would respond. He kept on keeping on, and his deeper mind never failed him.

▓

Ralph Waldo Emerson said, "All successful men have agreed in being 'causationists.' " Successful people, in other words, believe that their lives were not shaped by luck, but by law. Unsuccessful people believe in luck; successful people believe in cause and effect.

▓

Good luck is the reaction of your subconscious mind to your belief in good fortune.

▓

Those who believe that luck controls their destiny are ever waiting for something to turn up. They lie in bed, hoping that the mail carrier will bring them news of a legacy or that they have won a contest, sweepstakes, or lottery.

Luck relies on chance. Successful people rely on character, for character is destiny.

▓

The idea of competition engenders anxiety and excess tension. Don't be deterred from pursuing your goal by worries of competition. The truth is that the only competition you have is in your mind: between the thought of failure and the thought of success.

▓

Bless what you are doing now, realizing that it is a stepping-stone to your triumph and achievement.

Every thought is incipient action. When you begin to think of the riches within your subconscious mind and all around you, you will be amazed how successful ideas will flow to you from all sides.

The greatest discovery you can make is that there is an Infinite Power and Wisdom resident within you, and that this Power enables you to overcome all problems, rise above all hurdles, and handle life's tasks, and equips you with all the necessary attributes, qualities, and potential to make you a master of your fate and a captain of your soul.

Failure to acknowledge and unite with this Infinite Power and Wisdom within you will result in your relying on and being governed and controlled by events and conditions of the world. You will then tend to disparage *yourself* and exalt the power of circumstances, failing to realize the tremendous powers within you that could lift you up and set you on the high road to happiness, health, freedom, and the joy of living.

Align your thoughts and actions with God's Laws and you will rise triumphantly over problems, for "He never faileth."

Imagination is one of your greatest allies for success. Right now, you can look at an acorn and, with your imaginative eye, construct a magnificent forest full of rivers, streams, and rivulets.

You could people that forest with all kinds of life; furthermore, you could hang a bow on every cloud. Those who understand and use the laws of imagination find water in the desert and cause it to rejoice and blossom as a rose. They create cities where others see only a desert and a wilderness.

It is all right to have a dream, an ideal, or a goal, but you must have a solid foundation under your aspirations; otherwise they become idle fantasy, which wastes your energy and debilitates your entire organism. Castles built in the air without a basic knowledge of the powers of the subconscious to bring them into being are as inconsequential as whiffs of smoke.

Sadly, there are many men and women who do not understand this, and have not risen above their childhood daydreams.

Emerson said: "No one can cheat you out of ultimate success but yourself." Insist on the best in life; refuse the second best.

Believe you were born to succeed, and wonders will happen as you pray!

To give up your dreams is not to grow up; it is to start to die!

It is not fate that blocks your success or prosperity. It is you. Change your thought-life and keep it changed. Let your habitual thinking be on the idea of success and the knowledge that you can achieve whatever you conceive. *What things soever ye desire, when ye pray, believe that ye receive them, and ye shall have them.* (Mark 11: 24)

How much do you want what you want? Are you willing to leave your old ideas, the traditional view of things, and acquire new ideas, new imagery, and new viewpoints? Are you open and receptive? Are you willing to give up resentment and grudges over past failures?

If so, then there is no limit to the things you can achieve.

HOW HE FOUND SUCCESS

A brilliant young executive said to me, "I work very hard and put in long hours. My suggestions and recommendations to the management have been accepted and have made money for the organization. But I have been passed up for promotion the past three years. Even my subordinates have received increments and promotions."

This man was industrious and intelligent and apparently worked arduously. His inability to find the success he sought in his career was rooted in his relationship with his ex-wife.

For three years there had been litigation over division of their property, alimony, and child support. Subconsciously, he did not want to make any more money until the lawsuit was over, as he felt the more money he made, the more alimony the court would assess. He resented paying the temporary allowance granted by the court, feeling it was excessive, and he was waiting for final adjudication.

I explained to him the way his subconscious mind works, and that *he was actually decreeing that he didn't want any more money,* and that he had definitely emotionalized that negative concept. When you mentally wish to withhold wealth from another, you also automatically withhold it from yourself. This is why the Golden Rule tells you to think, speak, and act well toward your neighbor and never to indulge in hate, resentment, or carping criticism, for the simple reason that you are the only thinker in your universe, and your negative thoughts set up negative reactions in all departments of your life. Your subconscious mind is always fabricating and projecting on the screen of space the *totality* of your thought-life.

This young executive perceived that he had been blocking his own expansion and promotion. As we talked more, he came to understand that love casts out hate and that as he wished health, love, peace, and prosperity for his ex-wife and his children, he would attract to himself equally all these qualities. He also began to see that she was entitled to a reasonable sum of money for the support of his three children, that he should give it gladly, joyously, and lovingly, and that as he gave freely it would return multiplied. He began to frequently recite the following prayer:

> God is love, and God is life. This life is one and indivisible. Life manifests itself in and through all people; it is at the center of my own being. I know that light dispels the darkness; so does the love of the good overcome all evil. My knowledge of the power of love overcomes all negative conditions now. Love and hate cannot dwell together. I now turn the light of God upon all fear or anxious thoughts in my mind, and they flee away. The dawn (light of truth) appears, and the shadows (fear and doubt) flee away.
>
> I know Divine love watches over me, guides me, and

makes clear the path for me. I am expanding into the Divine. I am now expressing God in all my thoughts, words, and actions; the nature of God is love. I know that *perfect love casteth out fear.*

In a few weeks' time, an inner transformation took place in this young man, and he became amiable, affable, genial, and loving. He had a spiritual rebirth. His professional life immediately took a turn for the better, and he received a handsome promotion.

Techniques for Achieving Success

Here are five steps to achieving success.

Step 1: Find out the thing you love to do, then do it. Success is in loving your work.

Step 2: Have at heart those who seek your services. In your work, in other words, your motive must be altruistic. You must serve others, thereby casting your bread upon the waters.

Step 3: Specialize in some particular branch of work and know more about it than anyone else.

Step 4: Be sure that the thing you want to do does not seek out your success only. Your desire must not be selfish; it must benefit humanity. The path of a complete circuit must be formed; in other words, your idea must go forth with the purpose of blessing or serving the world. If what you desire is to benefit yourself exclusively, the circle or complete circuit is not formed, and you may experience a short circuit in your life, which may consist of limitation or sickness.

Step 5: Never forget the underlying power of the creative forces of your subconscious mind. Knowing that there is a mighty force in you that is capable of bringing to pass all your desires gives you confidence and a sense of peace. This is the energy in back of all steps in any plan of success.

You may say, "How can I put the first step of your steps to success into operation, if I don't *know* what my true place is or what I should do?" In such a case, pray for guidance as follows, knowing that the *idea of success* contains all the essential elements of success: "The Infinite Intelligence of my subconscious mind reveals to me my true place in life." Repeat this prayer quietly, positively, and lovingly to your deeper mind. As you persist with faith and confidence, the answer will come to you as a feeling, a hunch, or a tendency in a certain direction. It will come to you clearly and in peace, and as an inner silent awareness.

There is a law of mind that states that supply and demand are two aspects of one thing. What you are seeking is also seeking you. If you place your faith in Infinite Intelligence, it will direct you to your true place.

Affirm: Infinite Intelligence reveals to me my hidden talents and shows me the way I should go.

Affirm: I believe and accept without question that there is a creative intelligence in my subconscious mind that knows all and sees all. I know that I am directed rightly to my true place in life. I accept this inner guidance without question. I am here for a purpose, and I am willing to fulfill that purpose now.

Every night, still the activity of your mind and enter into a quiet, relaxed mental state. Gather all your thoughts together and focus all your attention on seeing your desired success as already a reality. Give all your attention to this mental image. Feel it. Experience it. See a newspaper article declaring it. Your steadied attention will create a deep, lasting impression on your subconscious mind.

※

Many people start a desirable project or begin pursuing a desirable goal, but then find that they are unable to follow through with it, stay with it, and complete it.

If you've ever had such an experience, it's likely that this attitude has become an expectation—that is, you know that something will come up and that you'll probably once again not be able to follow through with your intentions.

Learn that what you expect, you experience. You must, therefore, break this so-called jinx by boldly affirming the following before the commencement of any desired activity: "Infinite Intelligence is within me and knows how to complete all undertakings. If I waver or falter, I need only ask for and trust in the guidance of Infinite Intelligence, which is my own subconscious mind, and I will succeed."

※

Many highly successful people quietly affirm "success" over and over many times a day until they reach a conviction that success is theirs. They know that the *idea* of success contains all the essential elements of success. Likewise, you can begin now to repeat the word *success* to yourself with faith and conviction. Your subconscious mind will accept it as true of you, and you will be under a subconscious compulsion to succeed.

Go to sleep genuinely feeling and imagining success every night and feeling perfectly satisfied, and you will soon succeed in implanting the idea of success in your subconscious mind.

Principles to Remember and Apply

▶ There is no true success without peace of mind.

▶ Hold a picture in your mind of what you want to be and dramatize it in your imagination, knowing that your subconscious mind will develop it and bring it to pass. Remain faithful to this mental picture, and the way will open up and you will become that which you imagined and felt as true.

▶ A successful person cannot be selfish. His or her main desire in life must be to serve humanity.

▶ Repeat the word "Success" to yourself frequently with faith and conviction, and you will be under a subconscious compulsion to succeed.

▶ You were born to succeed, not to fail. The Infinite in you can't fail.

▶ No one can cheat you out of ultimate success but yourself.

▶ Good luck is the reaction of your subconscious mind to your belief in good fortune.

▶ A burning desire to be and to do will start you off on the high road to success and achievement. Identify yourself with your goal or desire by mentally and emotionally uniting with it. As you do this, Infinite Intelligence will activate the power of your subconscious mind and bring it to pass.

❯ When you condemn, criticize, demean, and belittle others, you are creating negative, counter-productive qualities within yourself.

❯ The word "sin" means to miss the mark. You are sinning against the Infinite Intelligence within you when you fail to lead a full, happy, prosperous, and successful life.

❯ Find out what you love to do, then do it. If you don't know your true expression, ask for guidance. Affirm frequently, "The Infinite Intelligence of my subconscious mind reveals to me my true expression."

❯ The only obstacle to your success and achievement is your own thought or mental image.

15 Your Unlimited Power for Self-Acceptance

Life created you for a purpose.

■

*B*less those around you, and you will discover that by blessing others, you too will be blessed, and all sense of personal lack will be overcome.

■

Honor and approve of the self within you. God dwells in you, and your self is the presence and power of God.

■

Know that you are wanted and loved because God wants you; that you are adequate to every task; that you are needed in the scheme of life; and that if you are not now, you soon can be fulfilling your role in the universe.

■

There is genius within you. Attune yourself with the Wisdom and Intelligence of your subconscious, and the genius in you will be revealed.

Inasmuch as you live with yourself all the time, it is of the greatest importance that you like yourself.

Unless you exalt the God-Self within you, you will feel inadequate and insecure, which contradicts both your deep psychological and spiritual necessity for self-esteem and God's will for you.

As Ralph Waldo Emerson often pointed out, the great so often appear great to us because we are, through self-denigration, so commonly on our knees.

Love of self, in the true biblical meaning, has nothing to do with egoism or self-aggrandizement. On the contrary, it is the wholesome veneration for the Divinity within you.

There is no such thing as an inferior or superior person. *Ye are gods; and all of you are children of the most High.* (Psalm 82:6)

▓

You have the power, ability, and capacity to do God-like things, for what is true of you is true of God. Think of all the wonderful things you can accomplish as you call on the Infinite Power within you, and you will set aside all the false beliefs and opinions you hold about your insignificant or lowly place in the world.

Behold, the kingdom of God is within you. (Luke 17:21) That is how important and wonderful you are!

▓

There are tremendous possibilities within you.

▓

Learn to accept forgiveness.

Forgive yourself for whatever failures and shortcomings you have in your past, for whatever ways you have not risen to your highest potential. Self-condemnation blocks the flow of cosmic energy into your life, robbing you of vitality, enthusiasm, and expansion in your life. It brings failure and misery. Self-forgiveness brings joy, happiness, and prosperity. Learn to forgive yourself.

▓

It is your sacred task, out of love for God—which ultimately means out of love for yourself—to positively and definitely refuse to accept anything less for yourself than peace of mind, your true place in life, abundance, and security.

You are here to discover your God-Self.

We rise as high as our dominant aspiration and descend to the level of our lowest concept of ourselves. Think kindly of yourself and have high hopes.

There are important reasons for you to accept yourself.

You are Life expressed. Life became you, and you are an instrument for Life's expression. You are very important, therefore, to Life, and you must recognize that Life is intensely interested in your welfare, development, and unfoldment, because you have a special work to do here.

Timidity is a state of mind. Do the things that you fear to do. Then the death of fear is certain, and you will find that you can lift yourself up to astonishingly great heights.

Remember these important truths:

Refuse to accept suffering and never resign yourself to any situation. The cause of all is your own mind and spirit, and as you are the only thinker in your universe, you can change your thoughts. Then, there is nothing that can defeat you.

Remember these things and you will find that you can lift yourself up mentally over all conditions and circumstances.

▦

Confidence means "with faith."

Your difficulties may be many, your obstacles challenging, your opposition rather formidable, but with Infinite Intelligence within you, you can move through the changes of life with a deep, unshakable, continuing confidence.

▦

The Creative Intelligence that made you never loses interest in that which It creates.

▦

Do not permit your feelings to unite with an image of limitation, as you will then generate the consequences of that unholy alliance. Stop focusing on your insufficiencies and lacks. They are not only a lie, they are a rejection of the Divine within you, and you demote your Self when you give them attention.

Approve of yourself; you are an individualized expression of God.

▦

You are a spiritual being, living in a spiritual universe, governed by a perfect God, operating under His perfect Divine law. Know this, and you will never feel inadequate. Your mind will be void of all self-doubt, worry, fear, and tension.

▦

You cannot manifest your good in a depressed state. Affirm and focus your attention on the Presence of God within you, and you will dissipate all the fearsome shadows lurking in your mind and rise above all obstacles, obstructions, and difficulties.

Don't let your problems weigh you down. You are here to discover the Divinity within. You are here to meet problems, difficulties, and challenges, and then to overcome them.

It is in overcoming obstacles that you develop character, and character is destiny.

If I could show you a nobler, sweeter, grander concept of yourself, do you think you could welcome and embrace it? It is right there inside of you, longing for your attention and care. It suffers from your neglect like an orphaned child, and you suffer as well.

Its name is your Greater Self, the God-Presence within you, and it has equipped you with almost illimitable possibilities of self-development.

No two people are alike, any more than any two leaves of a tree or two crystals of snow are alike. That is why *you* are here for a purpose, and it is not lowly.

Emerson said: "I am an organ of God and God hath need of me where I am, otherwise I would not be here."

If not being certain of your true place in life is what is holding you back from self-acceptance, call upon Infinite Intelligence within you to reveal to you your true place in life. Then follow the lead, which will come clearly and distinctly into your conscious, reasoning mind.

※

Within your subconscious you will find the answer to your most perplexing problems and the cause for every effect. There is an infinite healing presence in your subconscious that can heal your troubled mind and broken heart. The treasure-house of infinity is within you. It can free you from fear and from all kinds of material and physical thralldom and misery.

※

We all want to be what we want to be, do what we love to do, and have what we want to have. *You* can achieve all these goals in life, because you have been endowed with the qualities and faculties to do so.

※

Remember, Divine Intelligence responds to your habitual thinking. Therefore, think spiritual, noble, lofty, and God-like thoughts, and you will see the fallacy of lack of self-acceptance.

※

Do not waste your energy and vital substance by thinking about old misdeeds, failures in judgment, and any and all form of personal grievances. To do so is like opening a grave—all you find is a skeleton.

You are the artist, the weaver, the designer, and the architect of your life.

Whether you are rich or poor, you can look at the stars at night; you can look at the sunset; listen to the songs of the birds; become enraptured with the beauty all around you.

Begin, now, to contemplate God's beauty—and let riches flow through your thoughts, words, and deeds.

Life is a mirror that reflects back to us precisely that which we deposit in our minds. Look through the eyes of love and beauty, so you will see love, beauty, and the riches of the Infinite within you.

Those who find God within themselves lose their self-doubt, misery, and suffering.

Great numbers of men and women do not trust themselves; they demean and lower themselves. Your real Self is God—the Divine Presence residing in your subjective depths, governing your entire body, watching over you when you are sound asleep. It is the unseen power that moves your hands, enables you to walk and talk, and is ever ready to reveal to you everything you need to know.

All that is required of you is that you trust this Presence and Power. To do this, you need only turn in silence within yourself.

※

Monitor your self-talk constantly. There is a law of mind that responds to what you believe and decree yourself to be. Ideas are conveyed to the subconscious by repetition, belief, and expectancy, and are made manifest in your life. You cannot grow if your self-talk is negative.

HOW THEY LEARNED SELF-ACCEPTANCE

A young lady in a department store said to me, "I am nobody. I was born on the wrong side of the tracks. I did not get a good education." I explained to her that she could completely banish all sense of inferiority and self-rejection by changing her concept of herself and by knowing that conditions, experiences, and events in her life were effects, not causes.

She decided to banish all sense of inferiority by realizing the following truths: "I am a daughter of God. I am unique; there is no one in the entire world like me, because God never repeats Himself. God is my Father and I am His child. God loves me and cares for me. Any time I am prone to criticize or find fault with myself, I will immediately affirm: 'I exalt God in the midst of me.' God is now expressing Himself in a wonderful way through me. I radiate love, peace, and goodwill to all. I am one with my Father, and my Father is God. I know the real Self of me is God, and from this moment forward, I have a healthy, reverent respect for the Divinity within me, which created me and gave me breath and all things."

As she meditated on these truths, her insecurity and inferiority vanished. She found the riches within first, and then she found the riches of life on the screen of space. She began to imagine the kind of life she wished to have. She soon became acquainted with a customer in the store who was the answer to her dreams. Soon thereafter, they were married and they built a wonderful life together. She had been lifted out of a humdrum life, to one of purpose and satisfaction.

A business executive in Los Angeles told me that in 1929 he and his brother lost everything in the market crash. Each of them had been worth more than a million dollars. His brother committed suicide, saying that he had lost everything and that there was nothing to live for.

This business executive then told me that *he* said to himself, "I have lost money; so what? I have good health, a lovely wife, abilities, and talents. I'll make it again. God will guide me and open up a new door for me. I am going to make millions." He rolled up his sleeves and went out as a gardener and did odd jobs here and there. He accumulated some money, invested it in stocks, and saw them rise to fabulous heights. He gave advice to others, and they made a small fortune.

Remember: External circumstances, events, and conditions are effects. It is your thoughts that are the only cause. Don't deny your self-acceptance because of any circumstances, events, or conditions you are in. Your thoughts are your way out and toward riches.

Techniques for Growing through Self-Acceptance

Affirm: I am continually releasing the imprisoned splendor within me.

░

One of the most powerful times to banish self-doubt is prior to sleep, when you are in a sleepy, drowsy, relaxed state and there is an outcropping of your subconscious mind. Before you drift off to sleep, approve of yourself, accept yourself, realizing that you are an individualized expression of God. Affirm: "God dwells in me, walks and talks with me. God is guiding me now. I can do all things through the God-Power that strengthens me. If God be for me, who can be against me? There is no power to challenge God, and God watches over me in all my ways. I realize every problem is Divinely outmatched and I grapple courageously with every assignment, knowing that God reveals the answer. God loves me and cares for me."

░

Build into your subconscious mind the quality of good you desire by meditating every day upon that quality.

░

Whenever you feel weak, inadequate, nervous, or insecure, unite with the One Being, the Life Principle, that animates all things, and say, *"He restoreth my soul."*

░

Every time you stand in front of or pass a mirror, say with conviction:

"_____ [your name], you are absolutely outstanding, you are a tremendous success, you are full of faith and confidence, and you are immensely wealthy. You are loving, harmonious, and inspired. You are one with God, and one with God is a majority."

Continue this practice and you will be amazed at the many wonderful changes that will take place in your business, finances, circle of friends, and home life . . . to say nothing of how you will begin seeing yourself.

※

If God be for us, who can be against us? (Romans 8:31) This Bible verse is of prime importance to all who wish to attain self-confidence. It is considered by people to be one of the greatest and most profound statements in the Bible. I teach men and women to personalize the verse to read "If God be for *me*, who can be against *me*?" Many repeat these words before the mirror every morning for three or four minutes. They have told me that as this thought penetrated their minds, they knew they could overcome all obstacles. They had a spiritual experience accompanied by a feeling of victory.

Become mentally absorbed in the beauty and wisdom of the truth of these words so that their truth takes possession of you, and then you can live with confidence.

※

Here is the four-step plan for self-acceptance.

Step 1: Because the subconscious mind is amenable to suggestion and is controlled by the conscious mind, all negative patterns and doubts can be expunged by repeating positive affirmations three or four times a day in order to establish a habit of constructive thinking. Realize that no matter what the past experience may have been, these can be completely eradicated by feeding the subconscious mind with eternal verities and life-giving patterns of thought.

Step 2: Never condemn, demean, or demote yourself. The moment a thought such as "I'm no good," "A jinx is following me," "I'm unwanted," or "I'm nobody," comes to your mind, immediately reverse the thought by saying, "I exalt God in the midst of me."

Step 3: Imagine yourself being welcomed and accepted graciously and enthusiastically by others. Imagine and hear your superiors and coworkers congratulating you on a job well done. Above all, believe in your image and in its reality.

Step 4: Realize and know that whatever you habitually think upon and image must come to pass, for that which is impressed on your subconscious mind must be expressed on the screen of space as experiences, conditions, and events. Then think only of the good. *Whatsoever things are true, whatsoever things are honest, whatsoever things are just, whatsoever things are pure, whatsoever things are lovely, whatsoever things are of good report. If there be any virtue, and if there be any praise, think on these things.* (Philippians 4:8)

Affirm: I know that I can give only what I have. From this moment forward, I am going to have a wholesome, reverent, and deep respect for my real Self, which is God. I am an expression of God and God hath need of me where I am, otherwise I would not be here. From this moment forward, I honor, respect, and salute the Divinity within me. I am one with the Infinite.

Principles to Remember and Apply

▶ Begin to contemplate that God's beauty and riches flow freely through your thoughts, words, and deeds, and you will experience the results of your thinking.

▶ When you begin to realize that God hath need of you where you are and that you are loved, needed, and wanted, a complete transformation takes place: You begin to release the riches of the Infinite as love, goodwill, inner peace, and abundance.

▶ The only moment that matters is this moment. The past is dead. It has no power over you.

▶ You build self-acceptance by knowing that the God-Power in you is almighty.

▶ Know, believe, and practice aligning yourself mentally with the God-Presence within you, knowing that It will respond to you and take care of you all the days of your life.

▶ Whenever you're prone to denigrate or demean yourself, affirm: "I exalt God in the midst of me." As you make a habit of this, all sense of self-rejection and inferiority disappears.

▶ Every problem is Divinely outmatched; this is why you can lead a triumphant life.

▶ *If God be for us, who can be against us?* (Romans 8:31) Personalize this verse—If God be for *me*, who can be against *me?*— and you will overcome all self-doubt.

▶ Self-condemnation blocks the flow of cosmic energy into your life, robbing you of vitality, enthusiasm, and expansion in your life. It brings failure and misery. Self-forgiveness brings joy, happiness, and prosperity. Learn to forgive yourself.

▶ Carefully monitor your self-talk. The law of mind responds to what you believe and decree yourself to be. Ideas are conveyed to the subconscious by repetition, belief, and expectancy, and are made manifest in your life. You cannot grow if your self-talk is negative.

▶ There is genius within you. When you are in tune with the wisdom and intelligence of your subconscious, the genius in you will be revealed.

16 Your Unlimited Power to Change Your Life

You are transformed only one way, and that is by the transformation of your mind.

▦

Choose peace, Divine guidance, and right action in your life, and decree that "goodness, truth and mercy shall follow me all the days of my life: and I will dwell in the house of the Lord forever."

▦

Infinite Intelligence is only able to act *for* you by acting *through* you—through the choices you make.

▦

When you are fearful and worried and when you vacillate and waver, you are not thinking. True thinking is free from fear, because it is thinking from the standpoint of universal principles and eternal verities.

▨

When you learn to choose wisely, you will choose happiness, peace, security, joy, health, abundance, and all the blessings of life. You will enthrone the spiritual values and truths of God in your mind. You will busy your mind with these eternal verities until they become part of your consciousness in the same manner that nutrients become part of your bloodstream.

▨

The key to your health, wealth, prosperity, and success in life lies in your wonderful capacity to make choices.

▨

If you do not choose from the Kingdom of Heaven within you, which is the presence of God in your deeper mind, you will make decisions based on events, circumstances, and conditions around you. You will overlook the powers within you and will exalt the powers of circumstances.

Choose from the Kingdom of God within you, and move forward on the high road to happiness, health, freedom, and the joy of living the abundant life.

Choose you this day whom ye will serve.
(Joshua 24:15)

▨

You are here to choose. You are here to do your own thinking, reasoning, and choosing. You have volition and initiative. This is why you are an individual. Accept your Divinity and your responsibility and choose for yourself, make decisions for yourself; do not rely on others to know what is best for you. When you refuse to choose for yourself, you are actually rejecting your Divinity and your Divine prerogatives and you are thinking from the standpoint of a slave, a serf, and an underling.

Choose to be healthy, happy, prosperous, and successful. Your subconscious mind is subject to the decrees and convictions of your conscious mind, and whatever you decree (choose) convincingly shall come to pass.

*F*or as a man thinketh in his heart, so is he.
(Proverbs 23:7)

We are constantly being called upon to choose in this life. We choose one suit of clothes in preference to another; we choose our minister, doctor, dentist, home, wife, husband, food, and car. We choose the life we will lead and whether it is in harmony with the Infinite Intelligence.

What are you choosing in your life?

Remember, your whole life represents the sum total of your choices.

Feeling and emotion follow thought. Choose your thoughts wisely and create for yourself a rewarding emotional life.

※

Choose to believe that what is true of God is true of you; then, from this moment forward, the preponderance of your thought and expectancy will come from Him who giveth to everything: life, breath, and all things. Your mind and heart will be always open for the influx of God's riches now and forevermore.

※

You move from your old patterns of thought by dwelling on the way you want things to be.

※

Picture yourself as the person you want to be. Be faithful to the new image, and it will sink down to your subconscious mind, where it will gestate in the darkness, and after a while it will come forth in your experience as the joy of the answered prayer.

You will become a new person in God and go forward from glory to glory.

※

*B*e ye transformed by the renewing of your mind. (Romans 12:12)

You can change your whole life, if you really want to. You must give up resentment and ill will. Negative thinking must be supplanted by constructive thinking. Change your thoughts and keep them changed, and you change your destiny. You can transform your whole life!

All of us should begin to remove the old, accepted viewpoints, opinions, and false beliefs implanted in our minds when we were young and impressionable. The average person thinks and expresses the thoughts of dead people.

You do not ride a mule to go from one place to another like some of your grandfathers did; neither do you send a message by pony express. In the same way, you should not permit dead, superstitious beliefs to govern, rule, and manipulate your mind.

An emotion is always the working out of an idea in your mind. The way to overcome and discipline your unwanted emotions is not through repression or suppression. When you repress an emotion, the energy accumulates in your subconscious mind and remains snarled there. This occurs in the same manner as the pressure increases in a boiler when all the valves are closed and the heat of the fire is increased. In the end, there is a powerful explosion.

If you sincerely wish to transform your life and rid yourself of unwanted behaviors, you must watch what you think and maintain control over your mental images.

You can change your thoughts by choosing love over fear, goodwill over ill will, joy over sadness, and peace over disquiet. The instant you receive the stimulus of a negative thought, supplant it with the mood of love and goodwill. Fill your mind with love; then the negative thoughts cannot enter.

▩

The greatest tyrant is a negative or unkind idea that controls your mind and holds you in bondage.

If you are full of resentment toward someone or are possessed by a grudge, these emotions will exert an evil influence over you and will govern your actions in a way that will be very different from what you may desire: You will be unpleasant, cynical, and sour when you want to be friendly, affable, and cordial. You will find everything wrong, when you want to be healthy, successful, and prosperous.

To bring about the desired change in your life, sincerely accept ideas of peace and love in your mind, and the corresponding emotions will govern, control, and guide you accordingly.

▩

If you really want to bring about change in your life, you can do so. You will achieve it. Regardless of how unjustly you have been treated or what a mean scoundrel someone has proved to be, this will make no difference to you when you awaken to your mental and spiritual powers. You know what you want, and you will definitely refuse to let the thieves (thoughts) of hatred, anger, hostility, and ill will rob you of peace, harmony, health, and happiness. You cease to become upset by people, conditions, news, and events by identifying your thoughts immediately with your aim in life. Your aim is peace, health, inspiration, harmony, and abundance. Feel a river of peace flowing through you now. Your thought is the immaterial and invisible power. Choose to let it bless, inspire, and give you peace—and move you into the life you desire.

If you wanted to go from one place to another, you would have to leave the first place. In a similar way, if you want to be a new person, you must first leave behind your old fears, hates, grudges, jealousies, and the like. You must focus your attention on the concepts of harmony, health, peace, joy, love, and goodwill in order to enter into your desired new joy of living.

HOW SHE CHANGED HER WAYS OF ANGER

A woman who had attended several of my public lectures on the power of the subconscious mind sought me out before the next lecture. She introduced herself as Marina R., then said, "I've always had a terrible temper, since I was a little girl. And lately . . . well, my new neighbors are impossible. They play loud music late at night, they leave their garbage cans uncovered for animals to turn over and rummage through, and they laugh if I say a word of reproach."

"You must find their behavior very trying," I said.

"That's not the half of it!" she proclaimed. "But I've found a way to deal with the situation without blowing my top. I understand, after listening to your lectures, that I mustn't allow my anger and hatred to poison my subconscious mind."

"And what is this way you've found?" I asked curiously.

Marina laughed. "It depends on the weather," she said. "If it's a nice day, I go dig in the garden. As I work, I say aloud to myself, 'I am digging in the garden of God and planting God's ideas.' If the weather isn't so good, I get a bucket and a roll of paper towels and wash the windows. As I do, I say, 'I am cleansing my mind with the waters of love and life.' It works every time. Not only do I get over the temptation to become angry, but I put myself in a positive frame of mind *and* I get a few chores done!"

Techniques for Personal Change

If you have trouble maintaining a positive perspective, when you open your eyes in the morning, say to yourself, "I choose happiness today. I choose success today. I choose right action today. I choose love and goodwill for all today. I choose peace today."

Stand before a mirror and affirm: I am here because God is seeking expression through me. I am here to contribute beauty to the world. I am here because I am unique and God has need of me and my uniqueness.

Suppose you want to get rid of a destructive habit. Assume a comfortable posture, relax your body, and be still. Get into a sleepy state. In this sleepy state, say quietly, over and over again as a lullaby, 'I am completely free from _____ [the habit]; harmony and peace of mind reign supreme." Repeat this slowly, quietly, and lovingly for five or ten minutes morning and night. Each time you repeat the words, the emotional value becomes greater. When the urge comes to repeat the negative habit, repeat the above affirmation out loud. By this means you induce the subconscious to accept the idea, and a healing follows.

▓

Affirm: I am always poised, serene, and calm. *He that is slow to wrath is of great understanding, but he that is hasty of spirit exalteth folly.* (Proverbs 14:29)

Principles to Remember and Apply

▶ The key to your health, wealth, prosperity, and success is your capacity to choose. Choose whatsoever things are true, lovely, noble, and God-like. Choose thoughts, ideas, and images that heal, bless, inspire, dignify, and elevate your whole being.

▶ Your power to choose is your highest prerogative, enabling you to select from the infinite treasure-house within you all the blessings of life.

▶ When you choose harmony, peace, and right action in your life, believe that the Infinite Intelligence within you will back your choices. This knowledge will give you confidence in creating the life you desire and releasing yourself from any habit you wish to be free of.

▶ Never hesitate to make a choice. You are a volitional, choosing being, and to refuse to choose is actually to reject your own Divinity.

▶ God, or Infinite Intelligence, will do nothing *for* you except *through* the choices you make.

▶ You transform yourself, discipline your thoughts, feelings, and reactions to life, and think, speak, act, and respond from your Divine Center, or the God-Self within you.

➤ In order to transform yourself, you must purify your emotions through right thinking. Emotion follows thought.

➤ In order to become a new person, you must desire with all your heart to change your thoughts and keep them changed.

➤ Change your present thought and keep it changed, and you will change your character and your destiny—because character is destiny.

17 Your Unlimited Power to Nurture Relationships

Cease seeing others through eyes of lack and limitation; instead, realize that, like you, they are one with the Infinite.

■

Do not permit people to take advantage of you and gain their point by attacks of the heart. Be firm but kind, and refuse to yield. Appeasement never wins. Refuse to contribute to others' selfishness and possessiveness. Remember, do that which is right. You are here to fulfill *your* ideal and remain true to the eternal verities and spiritual values of life.

Give no one in all the world the power to deflect you from your goal, your aim in life, which is to express your hidden talents to the world, to serve humanity, and to reveal more and more of God's wisdom, truth, and beauty to all people in the world.

Remain true to your ideal. Know definitely and absolutely that whatever contributes to your peace, happiness, and fulfillment must of necessity bless all people who walk the earth.

All you owe the other, as Saint Paul says, is love—and love is *you*, fulfilling in *your* life the law of health, happiness, and peace of mind.

When we understand the creative law of our own minds, we cease blaming other people and conditions for making or marring our lives. We are aware that externals are not the causes and conditioners of our lives and experiences. We know that our own thoughts and feelings create our destiny. *For as a man thinketh in his heart, so is he.* (Proverbs 23:7)

Because your thoughts are creative, whatever you think about another you are creating in your own life and experience. Thus, you must never place obstacles and impediments in the pathway of others, or you will find impediments and obstacles in place in your own life.

Remember that anyone who helps you to attain your objectives is a messenger employed by your Deeper Cosmic Mind, to aid you in the unfoldment of the drama of your life.

One does not get upset or resentful toward a person who suffers from a congenital deformity. Likewise, one should not be disturbed because some people suffer from mental deformities— that is, twisted and disturbed mentalities. One should have compassion for them. Understanding their mental and emotional chaotic state, forgive them.

Be intolerant of false ideas, but not of people.

You must not try, through the use of any subtle mental influence of prayer, to bend another to your will. You must trust the infinite intelligence of your subconscious to bring what you desire in your life. You *can* get what you want in life through Divine Law and Order without infringing on the rights of others. Then there is no occasion for the use of mental coercion to try to influence others to do your bidding.

Realize that your work is a wonderful opportunity for you to serve other people.

When you were young, your parents warned you to keep away from bad company. If you disobeyed, you felt your parents' disapproval. In a somewhat similar manner, you must not walk down the dark alleys of your mind and keep the company of resentment, fear, worry, ill will, and hostility. These are the thieves of your mind. They rob you of poise, balance, harmony, and health, and manifest themselves in your relationships with others.

You have the freedom to make your own choices. Take a personal inventory of the contents of your mind; then choose thoughts of health, happiness, peace, and abundance, and you will reap fabulous dividends in all your relationships.

▨

Not every critical comment from another will be false. If another finds fault with you and these faults *are* within you, rejoice, give thanks, and appreciate the comments. This gives you the opportunity to correct the particular fault.

▨

*F*or with what judgment ye judge, ye shall be judged. (Matthew 7:2)

When you truly understand this teaching and the way your subconscious mind works, you will be careful to think, feel, and act right toward others.

This is one of the reasons for the application of the Golden Rule in human relations.

▨

Remember that negative criticism cannot hurt you without your consent. You cannot be hurt when you know that you are master of your thoughts, reactions, and emotions. Emotions follow thoughts, and you have the power to reject all thoughts that may disturb or upset you because they are not in accordance with the law of harmony.

Don't respond negatively to the criticism and resentment of others. Do not give attention to falsehoods others speak about you. To do so means that you have descended to a state of low mental vibration and become one with the negative atmosphere of the other. No matter what lies others may spread about you, they cannot hurt you unless you accept the thought mentally. The negative thoughts and statements of others have no power to create the things they suggest. Because others speak ill of you does not make it so. Your thought is creative. Refuse to transfer the creative power within you to others. You are the master of your own mind and should positively refuse to let others disturb you or manipulate your mind. The suggestions of others have no power to create the things they suggest. The power is in your own thought.

Identify yourself with your aim in life, and do not permit any person, place, or thing to deflect you from your inner sense of peace, tranquillity, and radiant health.

▓

Don't make comparisons. In comparing yourself with others, you are placing the other on a pedestal and denigrating yourself.

▓

The only way another can annoy you is through your own thought. When you get angry, for example, you have to go through four stages in your mind:

1. You begin to think about what the other person said,

2. You decide to get angry,

3. You generate an emotion of rage,

4. You decide to act, perhaps by talking back and reacting in kind.

As you see, this entire process takes place in your mind. This is a rather poignant example of how thought rules the world.

There *are* difficult people in the world. They are argumentative, uncooperative, cantankerous, cynical, and sour on life. Just remember that misery loves company.

When you are around such people, think love in your heart, and it will be so.

We are all interdependent. You may need a doctor, a lawyer, a psychologist, or a carpenter—and they, in turn, may need you. You may need a friend to comfort you in difficult times, and a friend may need you. We need each other. Let us remember, then, to lift up God in everyone and to see each person as that person ought to be seen: as a child of God, radiant, joyous, prosperous, and free.

Be careful of how you give to others. Never rob a person of the opportunity to grow and to advance. The young person who receives money and help too easily and too frequently finds it easier than self-discovery and self-propulsion. Constant assistance is destructive to another's character. Teach others where to find the riches of life, how to become self-reliant, and how to contribute their best to humanity, and they will never want a handout.

Give others the opportunity to overcome, and to discover their own characters. Otherwise, you will make them leaners.

Cease seeing others through eyes of lack and limitation; instead, realize that, like you, they are one with the Infinite.

Remember that all of us are part of humanity on the pathway of life.

Love is not possessiveness. Love is not jealousy. Love is not domineering or coercive. When you love another, your desire is to see the other happy, joyous, and free.

Love is freedom.

Honesty, sincerity, kindness, and integrity are also forms of love. Partners in love should be perfectly honest and sincere with the other.

It is not a loving relationship when one person joins in love with another for money, social position, or to lift up the ego.

You need not enter into a loving relationship with another for money, because if you understand and use the laws of mind correctly, you will never lack for wealth. Your wealth comes to you independently of anyone. You are not dependent on another for health, peace, joy, inspiration, guidance, love, wealth, security, happiness, or anything in the world. Your security and peace of mind come from your knowledge of the inner powers within you and from the constant use of the laws of your own mind in a constructive fashion.

░

A great mistake is to discuss your relationship problems with neighbors, relatives, or friends. Why cause numerous people to think negatively of your life or relationship? Moreover, as you discuss and dwell upon the so-called shortcomings of your loved one, you are actually creating these states within yourself. After all, who is thinking and feeling these ideas? You are! And as you think and feel, so are you.

Remember that difficulties will arise. No two human beings ever join their lives together or live beneath the same roof without clashes of temperament, periods of hurts and strain. But never display the unhappy side of your relationship to your friends. Keep your quarrels to yourself. Refrain from criticism and condemnation of your partner.

Remember, too, that any advice you receive that violates the Golden Rule, which is a cosmic law, is not good or sound.

░

In love and marriage, adjustments are needed, but this is not the same as trying to make your partner over. Such attempts only destroy the other's pride and self-esteem, and arouse a spirit of contrariness and resentment that proves fatal to the marriage bond.

░

Before you can draw to yourself the ideal partner and enter into a truly harmonious relationship, you must forgive the people in your past relationships.

Your resentment and hostility toward your previous partners becomes magnified in your subconscious mind and leads you over and over again to attract—and be attracted by—others who have an affinity with those negative feelings. It is the operation of the law of attraction. Like draws like. Birds of a feather really do flock together.

The key to changing this pattern is forgiveness. You must set yourself and your former partners free. You must replace your attitude of resentment with one of love and peace. If you can sincerely affirm, regarding your past partners, "I release you and let you go, wishing for you health, wealth, love, happiness, peace, and joy," you will find your whole understanding of love and marriage changed to a more spiritual basis.

HOW SHE FOUND THE RIGHT RELATIONSHIP

Rose L., a legal secretary in London, said to me during an interview, "I am in love with my boss. George is married and has four children, but I don't care. I've set my heart on him, and I will get him whatever it takes. As for his wife, that's her lookout, isn't it?"

Rose seemed perfectly willing to break up a home in order to gain her point. However, I explained to her that what she really wanted was not this married man. Her deepest desire was to have what she believed he and his wife had—a relationship in which each partner loved, cherished, and admired the other. "There is an ideal mate for you," I assured her, "one who is searching for you as hard as you search for him, and who will come to you without the encumbrance of an ongoing relationship with someone else. You can attract that mate to you, if you choose to."

"Why should I?" she demanded. "George is right there already. That's the man I want!"

"You may succeed in possessing this man," I replied. "You

may manage to bend him to your will. But you have no idea of the problems and difficulties you will be making for yourself. You will impregnate your subconscious mind with a sense of limitation and guilt. You know the commandment: *Thou shalt not covet thy neighbor's wife.* (Exodus 20:17) And the even greater commandment: *Whatsoever ye would that men should do to you, do ye even so to them.* (Matthew 7:12) These words give the entire law of a happy and successful life. In selfishness and greed, this is forgotten."

Rose suddenly saw the truth of what she was proposing to do and broke into sobs. Once she was quiet again, she agreed that she would want to attract an ideal companion without causing grief or pain to anyone else. She prayed by affirming: "I am now attracting a wonderful man who harmonizes with me spiritually, mentally, and physically. He comes to me without encumbrances and in divine order."

Shortly thereafter, Rose began to attend an art workshop. At one of these meetings, she met a young professor who turned out to be the man she really wanted. She discovered in this way that there is a law of mind that will bring to pass whatever she would accept as true.

Techniques for Building Healthy Relationships

Rearrange all your thoughts, imagery, and responses on the side of peace and harmony. If you see hatred in the other, practice knowing that your silent expression of God's love toward that person will dissolve everything unlike itself in the mind and heart of that person. This would be effective prayer, the truth that will set you free.

A wonderful spiritual prescription is to pray for all those with whom you associate, work, play, and love—wishing for them blessings of life. What you wish for others, you also attract to yourself.

▩

Realize that nobody acts in a contentious, hostile, antagonistic, and surly manner who is well-adjusted. There is a mental conflict somewhere in those who behave this way. There is something eating them inside. There is a psychic pain somewhere. Honor and salute the Divinity in that person: When you bless another, you will be identifying that person with God's qualities and attributes, remaining faithful to the God in that person. Radiate love and goodwill, being mindful that what is true of God is true of others as well as of you.

▩

If you find difficult people in your life, surrender them to God, declare your freedom in God, and let God take them under His care. You will then find yourself in green pastures and beside still waters.

▩

When you are in a quandary and are dealing with a difficult person or difficult people, write down, "This, too, will pass. There is a Divine and harmonious solution through the wisdom of my subconscious. I let go of all anger, resentment, and ill will now." Put this written prayer in a drawer marked "With God all things are possible." This is a symbolic way of releasing it, and it works wonders.

Affirm: "All the people who dwell in my mind are God's children. I am at peace in my mind with all the members of my household, wishing for all the same good I wish for myself."

Affirm: "I am the only thinker in the universe. I, alone, am responsible for what I think about. I refuse to give power to any person to annoy me or disturb me. I know that complaining about people and getting angry with them won't change them. I refuse to let anybody get under my skin. I bless them all and walk on."

Claim that your loved one is inspired from On High and is Divinely guided in all ways. To affirm this is one of the greatest motive powers for the demonstration of wealth in a relationship. All prosper because each is thinking of abundance.

Principles to Remember and Apply

- Show your deep appreciation for all those around you, members of your family and your coworkers. Give appreciation freely and lovingly.

- A hateful or resentful thought is a mental poison. Do not think ill of another, for to do so is to administer poison to yourself.

- The suggestions, statements, and actions of others cannot hurt you except through your mental participation. The creative power is in you. It is not what others say or do, it is your thought about it that matters.

▶ Your inner speech, representing your thoughts and feelings, is experienced in the reactions of others toward you and you toward them.

▶ Love is the answer to getting along with others. Love is respecting the divinity of the other.

▶ If another criticizes you, and these faults are within you, rejoice, give thanks, and appreciate the comments. This gives you the opportunity to correct the particular fault.

▶ Realize that in your work is an opportunity to serve other people. Claim that Infinite Intelligence reveals better ways in which you can serve.

▶ One of the things that could hold you back on your upward journey is to think you have a right to something that belongs to someone else. It is wrong to infringe on the rights of others. Wish for all what you wish for yourself.

▶ Never try to make another person over. These attempts are always foolish and destroy the pride and self-esteem of the other.

▶ It is a great mistake to discuss your relationship problems with neighbors, relatives, or friends. Why cause numerous people to think negatively of your life or relationship? Moreover, as you discuss and dwell upon the so-called shortcomings of your loved one, you are actually creating these states within yourself.

18 Your Unlimited Power to Obtain Healing

*If you were the richest person in the world, you
could not buy yourself a healthy body.
You can, however, gain health through the riches
of the mind.*

It is of great importance to point out that you can use the Universal
Healing Principle for any purpose. It is not confined to healing of
the mind or body. It is the same principle that attracts to you the
ideal husband or wife, helps you to prosper in business, finds for
you your true place in life, and reveals answers to your most difficult problems. Through the correct application of this principle,
you can become a great musician, physician, or diplomat. You can
use it to bring harmony where discord exists, peace where there is
pain, joy in place of sadness, and abundance in place of poverty.

The way to healing is already within you. You do not have to
beg, supplicate, or beseech God. All you have to do is change the
stream of your mental thought and imagery.

If, in praying for healing, you are constantly naming your aches and symptoms, you inhibit the release of the healing power and energy of your subconscious mind. Cease describing your symptoms and being completely engrossed and absorbed in your ailment, or you will make matters worse. Let your vision be on perfect health and vitality, and you will begin to release the Cosmic Power instantaneously. Train and discipline yourself to maintain the high vision. Chant the beauty of the good, and keep looking up. Affirm with deep understanding that the Infinite Intelligence that created your body is healing it. As this idea sinks into your subconscious mind, healing will follow.

Think of the healing, not the illness.

The Book of Proverbs says, *For as he thinketh in his heart, so is he.* (Proverbs 23:7) Your health is controlled very largely by the way you think all day long. By guiding your mind toward thoughts of wholeness, beauty, perfection, and vitality, you will experience a sense of well-being. If you dwell on thoughts of worry, fear, hate, jealousy, depression, and sorrow, you will experience sickness of mind, body, and affairs.

Cease talking about your worries and anxieties about world conditions, for that will only magnify your inner troubles and make your condition worse, because your mind always amplifies what it looks upon.

■

The body moves as it is moved upon; the body acts as it is acted upon.

■

The Infinite Healing Presence—the same Power and Energy that guides the planets and the stars in their courses and governs the billions of cells in your body—is always seeking an outlet through you. Trust It; believe in It. Realize that your body is basically spiritual substances, not just flesh and blood. Let this Power flow through you. Do not hinder It by fear and doubt.

■

We are told a wonderful story in the eighth chapter of Luke about a woman who had an issue of blood for twelve years, and who physicians could not heal. The Bible says she pressed through the multitude and touched the border of Jesus' garment and was made whole.

This means that the person who pushes his or her way through the "multitude" of culturally-acquired and family-acquired false opinions, false beliefs, and fears in his or her mind, which thwart healing, and brushes them all aside and gives himself or herself wholeheartedly to the Infinite Healing Presence, will receive a healing response. The woman in the Bible committed herself completely, trusting the Healing Presence unequivocally. And she was made whole.

Begin to use your mind in the right way now. Refuse to give

power to anything but the Healing Presence that is within you. Then you will be like the woman who succeeded in pushing her way through family and societal beliefs of lack, illness, and the like and mentally and emotionally touched the Presence of God, resulting in an instantaneous healing.

If you think that God wants you to be sick or through illness is testing you in some strange way, or if you think that God would create sickness, such a God is not worthy of your consideration and attention. The belief is only a false, superstitious concept in your mind. Remember always that the universal law of life is self-preservation, and in the Law of the Universe, there is only a principle of health, none of disease; only a principle of abundance, none of poverty; only a principle of honesty, none of deceit; only a principle of beauty, none of ugliness.

Your surgeon may remove the block, but unless you change your thinking, there will be no permanent healing.

A personal healing will ever be the most convincing evidence of your subconscious powers.

Nothing appears on your body except when the mental equivalent is first in your mind; as you change your mind by drenching it with healthy affirmations, you change your body.

All of us have heard the expression, "You are what you eat." We know that many physical and mental diseases can result from the lack of acquiring certain vitamins and chemicals in our diets. We know that there are dangers in consuming excessive quantities of fat, which interferes with the mechanical efficiency of all our vital organs, such as the heart, lungs, liver, and kidneys.

All this is important, but for your truly healthful living, your mental and spiritual diet is of the greatest importance.

The food that ultimately determines the healthful quality of your life is your thoughts. We have all known people who have had the choicest food and a perfectly balanced diet, according to the laws of nutrition, but still developed destructive and degenerative diseases.

Your habitual thinking nourishes and sustains your conditions and causes them to increase and magnify in your experience. Fear thoughts, worry and critical thoughts, and angry and hateful thoughts are the food of sickness, despondence, failure, and misery. When you feed your mind with negative food, sickness, lack, misery, and suffering come into your life.

The doctors who are treating you will do everything medical science can do. But you can do more. You can make a conscious decision to become more at ease with yourself.

Sometimes we are told that a particular person is a "natural-born healer." This is superstition. The truth is that we are all natural-born healers. The Healing Presence of God is within all of us. We can all contact it with our thoughts, and it will respond to us.

Anyone can set the law of healing into operation, just the same as anyone can learn to drive an automobile. Learn the laws of mind and the ways of the Infinite Intelligence within you; the Infinite Healing Presence responds to your thoughts and to your beliefs.

The prayers of the healer who lays a hand on another are simply appealing to the cooperation of the patient's subconscious. If you issue prayers of equal conviction to your subconscious, it will likewise become impregnated with the idea of health, and a healing response will take place. For according to your faith is it done unto you.

▦

There is a miraculous healing power within you for which no healing is too great. There is no great or small in the God that made us all; there is no big or little, no hard or easy.

▦

Do not give power to the ailment or condition. Give power and allegiance to the Infinite Healing Presence.

Learn to let go and relax. Realize that the Creative Intelligence that fashioned your body and started your heart can heal its own handiwork. Be assured that this infinite Healing Presence is instantly available. You can always draw on its power through the creative law of your own mind. Make use of this power now and bring about healing in your life, for *with God all things are possible.* (Matthew 19:26) *I will restore health unto thee, and I will heal thee of thy wounds, saith the Lord.* (Jerermiah 30:17)

What is it that heals? Where is this healing power? The answer is that this healing power is called by many names, including Nature, Life, God, Creative Intelligence, Cosmic Consciousness. But by whatever name, the healing power resides in the subconscious mind of each person. It is the only healer there is. Since your childhood, it has been healing the cuts and bruises on your body. It knows exactly how to do it, without your conscious effort or knowledge of how.

According to your faith be it unto you. (Matthew 9:29) There is only one process of healing and that is faith; there is only one healing power: your subconscious mind.

You do not have to belong to any particular religion in order to use and participate in this healing process. Your subconscious will heal the burn or cut on your hand even though you profess to be an atheist or agnostic.

There is only one Universal Healing Principle operating through everything: the cat, the dog, the tree, the grass, the earth. In most of life, this Principle operates as innate instinct. We humans are the only forms of life who are aware of this life principle and can consciously direct it to bless ourselves in many ways.

Scientists inform us that all the cells in our body are replaced every eleven months. You can heal disease, then, by refusing—as your body is rebuilding itself—to build defects back into your body through thoughts of fear, anger, jealousy, and ill will. Continually affirm your faith in the healing power of the Infinite Intelligence within you and increase the inflow and distribution of the vital forces of your subconscious mind throughout your system.

⬛

Eliminate thoughts of fear, worry, anxiety, jealousy, hatred, and every other destructive thought, as they tend to tear down and destroy your nerves and glands, the very body tissues that control the elimination of all waste material—including the wasteful thoughts of fear, worry, jealousy, and the like.

⬛

It is abnormal to be sick; it simply means you are going against the stream of life and thinking negatively. The instinct of self-preservation is the strongest instinct of your nature, and it constitutes a most potent, ever-present, and constantly operative truth, inherent in your nature.

⬛

The law of life is the law of growth; all nature testifies to the operation of this law by silently, constantly expressing itself in the law of growth. Where there is growth, there is life; where there is life, there is harmony; and where there is harmony, there is perfect health.

If your thought is in harmony with the creative principle of your subconscious mind, you are in tune with the Innate Principle of Harmony. If you entertain thoughts that are not in accordance with the Principle of Harmony, these thoughts will cling to you, harass you, worry you, and finally bring about disease.

▓

Whatever medical problems your doctor uncovers will be made worse as long as you allow your subconscious mind to be saturated with the negative statements about your health by yourself or others. If you find yourself becoming beset with doubts, remind yourself that the Creator can correct Its creation.

▓

You can pray healingly for another. This is sometimes called "absent healing." You are not trying to send out thoughts to another. Your treatment is just a conscious movement of thought: As you focus on and become conscious of the qualities of health, well-being, and relaxation, these qualities will be resurrected in the experience of the person you seek to heal, and results will follow.

In reality, there is in fact no actual "absent treatment," as opposed to present treatment. As there is no time or space in the mind principle, Infinite Mind, or Intelligence, is present in its entirety at every point simultaneously. It is never absent from anywhere.

▓

In the Book of Ecclesiasticus, Chapter 38: 1-15, we read these words:

Honour physicians for their services, for the Lord created them; for their gift of healing comes from the Most High, and they are rewarded by the king. The skill of physicians makes them distinguished, and in the presence of the great they are admired. The Lord created medicines out of the earth, and the sensible will not despise them. By them the physician heals and takes away pain; the pharmacist makes a mixture from them. God's works will never be finished; and from him health spreads over all the earth.

My child, when you are ill, do not delay, but pray to the Lord, and he will heal you. Give up your faults and direct your hands rightly, and cleanse your heart from all sin. . . . Then give the physician his place, for the Lord created him. There may come a time when recovery lies in the hands of physicians, for they too pray to the Lord that he grant them success in diagnosis and in healing, for the sake of preserving life. He who sins against his Maker, will be defiant toward the physician.

God has created the physician just as God has created you. If you pray for health and you have the conviction of the Presence of God where the trouble is, then *he will heal you.* However, when you find that you cannot heal an illness or grow a tooth or mend a broken bone *at once* through prayer, *then give the physician his [or her] place.* This is common sense and certainly much better than being a cripple for life.

※

Do you really believe the God Presence can heal you now? Do you believe implicitly in the Infinite Healing Presence within you, or do you think disease is independent of your mind? Do you think you are incurable? Do you think the will of God for you is sickness, pain, and trouble? If so, these thoughts of impotence, sickness, and suffering are robbing you of health, vitality, and peace of mind. False ideas have no power other than the power you give them.

Open your mind and heart to the healing power of God, and the healing power will flow into you as surely as the light and heat of the sun will come into your habitation when it is thrown open to receive the light and heat.

※

A bottled-up emotion repressed in the subconscious will sooner or later be translated into a bodily symptom.

HOW THEY ACHIEVED HEALING

In November 1966, I gave a series of lectures at the New Orleans Unity Society in New Orleans. One of the men present told me that some months previously he had been crippled with arthritis and was unable to bend his knees. One evening a holdup man came in to the store where he was working, pointed a gun at his head, and said, "Kneel down behind the counter!" He replied, "I can't. I'm crippled with arthritis." The bandit said, "I'll give you ten seconds to kneel down or I'll kill you!" The man told me, "I bent my knees easily! Since then, I have gradually gotten much better. My doctor says that the calcareous deposits are all gone, and the suppleness and mobility of my joints have returned. How do you account for it?"

This is a good question.

I explained to him that there was a principle of healing involved there and that if he had understood the principle and applied it, he could have been healed prior to the holdup. As he was able to bend his crippled knees at the point of the pistol, it stands to reason that the power to bend his knees, to walk, and to run was always present within him—even though he believed otherwise. What had occurred was this: Quite obviously, the pistol had no power to heal. The man had been crippled for several years, he said, unable to bend his knees. All his attention and vision, therefore, were bound up in his pain, aches, limitation, and physical handicap. Suddenly, however, when this robber entered the store, the man's attention was taken off his ailment, and his vision was directed to saving his life at all costs, as self-preservation is the first law of life. Immediately, he released the miraculous healing power that neutralized and dissolved everything unlike itself. He was healed by the Cosmic Power within him.

The Cosmic Power is always available to us, but our fears, false beliefs, and misbegotten concepts hold us in bondage.

In his book, *Suggestive Therapeutics*, Hippolyte Bernheim expounded on the fact that the suggestion of the physician to the patient was exerted through the subconscious mind.

Bernheim stated that he produced a blister on the back of a patient's neck by applying a postage stamp and suggesting to the patient that it was a fly-plaster.

Dr. M. Bourru put a subject into the somnambulistic condition and gave him the following suggestion: "At four o'clock this afternoon, after the hypnosis, you will come into my office, sit down in the armchair, cross your arms upon your breast, and your nose will begin to bleed." At the hour appointed the young man did as directed. Several drops of blood came from the left nostril.

As a man thinketh in his heart [subconscious mind] *so is he.*

In the healing of the body, it is *desirable* to secure the concurrent faith of both the conscious and subconscious mind. However, this is not always essential. The faith required in the healing of any problem is a purely subjective faith, and it is attainable upon the cessation of active opposition on the part of the objective or conscious mind. As long as you allow yourself to enter into a state of passivity and receptivity by relaxing the mind and the body and getting into a sleepy state, your passivity will become receptive to subjective impression.

For example, I was once asked by a man, "How is it that I got a healing through a minister? I did not believe what he said when he told me that there is no such thing as disease and that matter does not exist."

This man at first thought his intelligence was being insulted, and he protested against such a palpable absurdity. The explanation is simple. He was quieted by soothing words and told to get into a perfectly passive condition, to say nothing, and think of nothing for the time being. His minister also became passive, and affirmed quietly, peacefully, and constantly for about half an hour that this man would have perfect health, peace, harmony, and wholeness.

In the man's quiet, receptive state, the suggestions of perfect healthfulness by the minister were easily conveyed to and accepted by the man's subconscious mind. The subjective minds of the man and the minister were then in rapport.

The minister was not handicapped by doubting, antagonistic autosuggestions of the patient, and in his sleepy, drowsy state, the man's conscious mind's resistance was reduced to a minimum. The subconscious mind of the man, being controlled by suggestion, exercised its function, and a healing followed.

During a visit to San Francisco some months ago, I visited a friend in a hospital. He had a kidney infection and also a damaged heart. He said to me, "I won't be here long. I am constantly picturing myself back at my desk at my office and in my home with my loved ones. I am doing all the things in my mind that I would do were I whole and perfect. It is my divine right to be healthy, and my vision is always on being well. I have an intense desire to be well and stay well, and I will be well."

Even though his doctors had told this man he would need a lengthy hospital stay of several weeks, he was in the hospital only ten days.

You must want to be well with all your heart and soul, and then you will be well and stay well, also.

While giving a lecture at the Yoga Forest University in Rishi-kesh, India, some years ago, I chatted with a visiting surgeon from Bombay. He told me about Dr. James Esdaille, a Scotch surgeon, who worked in Bengal before ether or other modern methods of anesthesia were discovered. In the 1840s, Dr. Esdaille performed about four hundred major operations of all kinds, such as amputations and removal of tumors as well as operations on the eye, ear, and throat. All operations were conducted under mental anesthesia only. This Indian doctor at Rishikesh informed me that the postoperative mortality rate of patients operated on by Dr. Esdaille was extremely low, probably two or three percent. Patients felt no pain, and there were no deaths during the operations.

Dr. Esdaille suggested to the subconscious minds of all his patients, who were in a hypnotic state, that no infection or septic condition would develop. You must remember that this was before Louis Pasteur, Joseph Lister, and others who pointed out the bacterial origin of disease and causes of infection due to unsterilized instruments and virulent organisms.

This Indian surgeon said that the low mortality rate and the general absence of infection, which was reduced to a minimum, was undoubtedly due to the suggestions of Dr. Esdaille to the subconscious minds of his patients. They responded according to the nature of his suggestion.

Donald L. is the author of a wonderful book on nutrition. It is quite scientific and very sound. However, he himself suffers from acute ulcers. His physician tried to treat his condition with antibiotics, linked with a special diet, but the ulcers only worsened.

When Donald described his situation in a conversation with me, I asked, "Have you noticed anything in your mental or emotional life that seems to be connected to the ulcers?"

He replied, "Not at all. But I'll tell you one thing. I can't pick up a newspaper or watch a newscast without feeling a pang. All the top stories are about suffering, crime, injustice, and inhumanity. It makes me livid. I spend several hours a week writing letters and e-mails to people in Congress and the government, telling them exactly what I think about their actions."

"I take it you don't think very highly of them," I said dryly. "Would it be fair to call these angry messages?"

"Certainly," Donald said, "and every bit of my anger is justified."

"Even the part that is responsible for your illness?" I asked. "You know, when you allow negative energy to build up inside yourself, it has an effect, even if you discharge much of it on an external target. If you want to be cured of your stomach condition, you will have to change your mental and emotional diet."

By the end of our talk, Donald had committed himself to adopting a new mental regimen:

"I am going to transform all negative impressions that come to me during the day. From now on, I will never permit news, propaganda, criticism, or negative statements of others to promote negative reactions in me. When I am tempted to react negatively and vindictively, I will stop immediately and affirm to myself boldly, 'God thinks, speaks, and acts through me now. His river of peace floods my mind and heart, and I am identified with my aim, which is peace and harmony.'"

This new way of reacting became a habit, and he had a remarkable healing in a short period of time.

Techniques for Achieving Healing

The following is a perfect example of what is sometimes called "absent treatment." A listener of our radio program in Los Angeles prayed as follows for her mother in New York, who had a coronary thrombosis: "The healing presence is right where my mother is. Her bodily condition is but a reflection of her thought-life, like shadows cast on the screen. I know that in order to change the images on the screen I must change the projection reel. My mind is the projection reel, and I now project in my own mind the image of wholeness, harmony, and perfect health for my mother. The infinite healing presence that created my mother's body and all her organs is now saturating every atom of her being, and a river of peace flows through every cell of her body. The doctors are divinely guided and directed, and whoever touches my mother is guided to do the right thing. I know that disease has no ultimate reality; if it had, no one could be healed. I now align myself with the infinite principle of love and life, and I know and decree that harmony, health, and peace are now being expressed in my mother's body."

She prayed in the above manner several times daily, and her mother had a most remarkable recovery after a few days, much to the amazement of her specialist.

Do not weaken your healing thoughts by saying such words as, "I wish I might be healed," or "I hope so." Know that health is yours. Keep in mind that how you *feel* about your prayer is "the boss." Become a vehicle for the infinite healing power of the subconscious mind. Pass on the idea of health to your subconscious mind to the point of conviction. Then relax. Through relaxation you impress your subconscious mind, enabling the kinetic energy behind the idea to take over and bring it into concrete realization.

The ideal way to practice spiritual mind healing—either for yourself or for another—is to completely withdraw all thought from symptoms and from the condition altogether. Whatever part of your or another's body you're praying about, do not think of this part as diseased. This would not be spiritual thinking. To think of a damaged heart or high blood pressure tends to suggest more of what you already have. Stop dwelling on symptoms, organs, or any part of the body. Turn your mind to God and His love. Feel and know that there is only one Healing Presence and Power, and that there is no power to challenge the action of God.

Think of yourself or the person for whom you are praying as a purely spiritual being. In other words, identify with the Spirit or Healing Presence within yourself or the other, claiming that what is true of the Spirit is true of yourself or the person you are trying to help. Then quietly and lovingly affirm that the uplifting, healing, strengthening power of the Healing Presence is flowing through you, making you whole. Know and feel that the harmony, beauty, and life of God manifest in you as strength, peace, vitality, beauty, wholeness, and right action. Get a clear realization of this, and the diseased condition will dissolve in the Light of God's love.

A Protestant minister I knew in Johannesburg, South Africa, told me the method he used during an illness to convey the idea of perfect health to his subconscious mind. His technique, as given to me in his own handwriting, is exactly as follows: "Several times a day I would make certain that I was completely relaxed mentally and physically. . . . After about five minutes I would be in a drowsy state, and then I affirmed the following truth: 'The perfection of God is now being expressed through me. The idea of perfect health is now filling my subconscious mind. The image God has of me is a perfect image, and my subconscious mind recreates my body in perfect accordance with the perfect image held in the mind of God.' " This minister had a remarkable healing.

◼

Another wonderful way to convey the idea of health to your subconscious is through disciplined or scientific imagination. I told a man who was suffering from sciatica to make a vivid picture of himself walking around in his office, touching the desk, answering the telephone, and doing all the things he ordinarily would do if he were healed. I explained to him that this idea and mental picture of perfect health would be accepted by his subconscious mind.

He lived the role and actually felt himself back in the office. He knew that he was giving his subconscious mind something definite to work upon. His subconscious mind was the film upon which the picture was impressed. After several weeks of frequent conditioning of the mind with this mental picture, the man was able to resume his normal life.

◼

*S*ay in a word, and my servant shall be healed.
(Luke 7:7)

You can pray healingly for another. Here's how:

Step 1: Feel the Presence of God—which is the presence of harmony, health, and peace—in your friend, going through and around him or her; feel that he or she is Divinely watched over.

Step 2: Even though the other person may not know about it, personally accept that the healing is taking place now, and that you sincerely believe it.

You can do this several times a day, if you wish. The healing may come slowly or it may come quickly, according to your belief.

⬛

During times of emotional or physical illness, affirm regularly and daily: I was created by the Infinite Intelligence in my subconscious mind. It knows how to heal me. I give thanks for the healing I know is taking place now.

⬛

Affirm: "God is healing me now."

Principles to Remember and Apply

▶ There is only one process of healing and that is faith. There is only one healing power—namely, your subconscious mind.

▶ Your subconscious, the builder of your body, is on the job twenty-four hours a day. You interfere with its life-giving patterns by negative thinking. Feed your subconscious with thoughts of harmony, health, and peace, and all the functions of your body will be normal.

▶ It is foolish to believe in sickness or something that can hurt or harm you. It is normal to be healthy. It is abnormal to be ill. There is within you an innate Principle of Harmony. Believe in perfect health, prosperity, peace, wealth, and Divine Guidance.

▶ Have faith in the Healing Power. If you have an illness or disease, imagine and feel that you are now doing all the things you would do if you were made whole.

▶ People may say it's impossible, but with God all things are possible. God, who created you, can heal you.

▶ If you believe something, it will be manifest whether or not you are consciously thinking of it. Therefore, believe only in that which heals, blesses, and inspires you.

▶ All of us are natural-born healers, because the Infinite Healing Presence is within us and we can contact it with our thoughts and beliefs.

▶ Food for the body is important, but your mental and spiritual diet is of supreme importance. The food that ultimately determines the healthful quality of your life is your thought. You are what you eat psychologically and spiritually.

▶ When you are sick and when you pray, if you do not get results immediately, go and see a doctor at once. Bless your doctor while you are continuing to pray for health and harmony.

▶ When praying, do not identify with the ailment or any part of the anatomy. Instead, affirm that the Infinite Healing Presence is flowing through you as harmony, health, peace, and joy.

▶ Negative and destructive emotions snarl up in the subconscious mind and are the cause of many diseases.

▶ The key to rapid recovery from sickness is to picture the ailment as temporary; then have a vivid picture of yourself back at your usual work. You can recondition yourself to health and harmony as you meditate frequently on harmony, vitality, wholeness, beauty, and perfection.

▶ You can't get something for nothing. The price you pay for healing is faith in the Infinite Healing Presence, for *according to your faith is it done unto you.*

▶ All healing takes place according to the belief of the individual. The subconscious mind is the creative medium; it is the builder of your body and the healer of the body. Whatever the conscious mind impresses on the subconscious, the latter faithfully reproduces. Lull yourself to sleep every night with the idea of perfect health, and your subconscious, being your faithful servant, will obey you.

▶ We did not create ourselves. Infinite Intelligence created us, and it can heal and restore us. Trust it, believe it, and call upon it, and you will get a response. Don't pretend to believe, but know in your heart that the creative intelligence that made all your organs knows how to heal and restore. According to your faith will it be done unto you.

19 Your Unlimited Power to Obtain Guidance

There is guidance for each of us, and by listening,
we shall hear the right word.

▦

A man's foes shall be they of his own household.
(Matthew 10:36)

The *household* is your state of mind. Your ability to truly receive guidance is related to your ability to achieve victory over the *foes* (negative thoughts) that would have you disbelieve.

▦

Everyone is a part of the One Mind. Guidance, therefore, may come unexpectedly into your life from others, who are acting then as messengers on behalf of your Deeper Cosmic Mind.

▦

Your Cosmic Power stands ready and waiting for your use, in the same way that the tap in your kitchen stands ready to give you water. Just as you have faith that when you turn on the tap water will flow, you must learn to expect answers and to have faith in Divine right action in all your undertakings. Do this, and ways will be wondrous beyond your imaginings.

※

Don't fall into the trap of so many: In spite of their statements of belief in their Higher Self, many are still trying to solve all of their problems on a conscious level. Intellect cannot solve all of the problems with which you are faced.

※

You have the perfect right to seek Infinite Guidance for bringing any good into your life, provided your motive is unselfish and your desire for health, happiness, peace, love, and abundance cannot possibly harm anyone. The Infinite Presence will aid you if what you are seeking is consistent with integrity and honesty.

If your thought *is* right—it conforms to the Golden Rule and the law of goodwill for all and it is not contradicted by thoughts of uncertainty and doubt—a feeling of inner peace and tranquillity wells up within you, assuring you that Divine Guidance is already working on your behalf.

※

There is a Principle of Right Action in the universe. The Cosmic Intelligence within you will give you anything you claim, feel, and believe. The Cosmic Mind has billions of channels through which to pour out its infinite blessings. You are a channel of God. Accept your good now.

When you have tried every conceivable way to solve a problem, and when you have sought counsel and expert advice from spiritual and other appropriate, knowledgeable sources, then do as Saint Paul suggests: "Having done all, I stand." Stand firmly on the truth that *your motivation is right* and that the Cosmic Power within you knows the answer and will reveal the perfect solution as you completely surrender the matter to God, knowing and believing in your heart that the answer will come. Then the day breaks and the shadows flee away.

The Universal Life Force, which is God in you, can inspire you and reveal to you everything you need to know. All you have to do is open your mind and your heart to receive.

You are immersed in and surrounded by an Infinite Presence that possesses the answers to all the difficulties and problems of the world and responds to your thoughts, this Presence is referred to as Omniscience, Omnipresence, Omnipotence, and Omniaction.

Omniscience is "all wisdom," that which knows all and sees all. This All Wise One created the whole world and the galaxies in space, and also created you. Being All Wisdom, It knows the answer to any problem under the sun.

Omnipresence is "all present," or "everywhere present," that which is within you and all around you: everywhere. There is no place that it isn't, that it cannot be. There is no answer to your request for guidance that it cannot have before it.

Omnipotence is "all powerful." This resource possesses the power and energy in the entire universe to bring guidance to you.

Omniaction is "all action." The Supreme Wisdom initiated all the activity in the entire universe: all cycles of time as well as rotation of earth and planets. Its principles and laws move rhythmically, harmoniously, systematically, and ceaselessly, governing the entire cosmos. It can put into action whatever activity or activities are necessary to bring into your life your means of guidance.

This incredible resource of Power or Energy is within you; it is present wherever you are. It makes no difference how many individuals this Energy is flowing through; there is always an inexhaustible supply, as It is the Infinite Source of all Energy. You can consider yourself the recipient of all the riches, power, and wisdom of the Infinite, and at the same time you deprive no one else of anything. Enthrone these truths in your heart and mind, and you will know the amazing resource that is ever available to you for guidance, at all times and in all ways.

You can meet any challenge because there is a Wisdom and Power within you that will enable you to overcome the problem. Realize that your difficulty or problem is a marvelous opportunity for you to demonstrate and prove to yourself your capacity to overcome; that you have Divine Guidance on your side.

▨

God is always successful in all His undertakings, and what is true of God is true of you, because you are heir to all His riches. It is your sacred task, therefore, to positively and definitely refuse to accept anything less than success in meeting your challenges. Keep on asking and knocking until your answer comes.

▨

It is through difficulties and problems that we discover our Divinity.

▨

No matter what the problem is, as you think about a Divine solution and the happy ending, you will find a subjective wisdom within you responding to you and revealing to you the perfect plan and showing you the way you should go.

▨

In ancient times and even to the present time, when royalty traveled, couriers and messengers were sent forth to prepare and get everything in readiness. A royal welcome was assured. Likewise when a nation's leader goes on a trip, special agents go over the route and keep a watchful eye at all times. No thieves, robbers, or gangsters—no harm—can come near royalty or national leaders as they travel, because of all the precautions taken for their safety.

Similarly, accept for yourself that Divine love and guidance go before you, and you will know that as you move through life, *every mountain* (problem) *and hill* (obstacle or difficulty) *shall be made low: and the crooked* (the ups and downs of life; the swings of fortune) *shall be made straight, and the rough places plain.* (Isaiah 40:4)

※

You are the victor in all circumstances, because God dwells in you. Therefore, every problem you face is Divinely outmatched.

※

Look for your guidance from the secret dwelling place of Infinite Intelligence within you, not from the external conditions, events, or circumstances, and you will not fail nor be disappointed.

※

When you're looking for help in some situation, know that what you are seeking is seeking you—that is, what you have a need to sell, someone has a need to buy; what you have a need to acquire, someone has the need to rid himself or herself of or give away. This will fill you with confidence, faith, and security that you have guidance in all your ways.

※

The solution lies within the problem. The answer is in every question.

Stand up to your problems; have a firm conviction in the Infinite Intelligence within you to solve them. The door will open, and the way will be shown to you.

When you say, "There is no way out; I have no chance; I'm all mixed up and confused; why don't I get an answer?" then you are listening to the winds of confusion, fear, and human opinion. But when you remember that there is a Spiritual Power within you—All-Wise and All-Knowing—you will have faith that there *is* a way out, and that it will be revealed to you. You need only give your subconscious the request, and you will attain its cooperation.

The answer to your prayer for guidance will not always come in a day. Trust, though, that Divine Guidance *will* bring about the answer in Divine Order and that there will be a happy solution, and that using this knowledge to control your thoughts and emotions, you can persevere with equanimity, regardless of your external circumstances. All you have to do is believe in the Divine Presence within you and trust in It. Wonders will happen in your life.

When you are seeking and picturing guidance and advancement, and the opportunity for more money and increased status and prestige is presented to you, then even if this opportunity is not the solution you anticipated, if you feel receptive to the idea, take it, and it will prove to be a step toward greater and grander opportunities.

*D*raw nigh to God, and he will draw nigh to you. (James 4:8)

This means that Infinite Intelligence is responsive to you and will answer when you call.

▩

Look within. If you look outside for help, you are denying the riches of God within and you are stealing power, wisdom, and intelligence from yourself.

▩

If you don't use your physical muscles, they will inevitably atrophy. You have mental and spiritual "muscles" that must also be exercised. If your thoughts, attitudes, motivations, and reactions are not God-like, your contact with God is broken. When a challenge then arises in your life, you will lack the certitude of faith in the right action of the outcome, and you will be fearful.

▩

The Infinite Intelligence deep in your subconscious mind is responsive to your request for guidance. You will recognize Its response as an inner feeling, an awareness, an overpowering hunch leading you to the right place at the right time, putting the right words into your mouth, and causing you to do the right thing in the right way.

▩

There are two reasons why you may not acknowledge your inner guidance: tension and failure to recognize the lead when it comes. If you are in a quiet, confident mood, you will recognize the flashes of intuition that come to you. Moreover, you will feel under a subjective compulsion to carry them out.

It is necessary, therefore, to be still and relaxed when you pray for guidance. Nothing can be achieved by tenseness, fear, or apprehension. Your subconscious mind answers you when your conscious mind is still, receptive, and relaxed.

*C*hoose you this day whom ye will serve. (Joshua 24:15)

The key to gratification in seeking guidance lies in your capacity to seek guidance in the direction of health, happiness, peace of mind, and abundance in your life. When you learn to think right, you will cease choosing pain, misery, poverty, and limitation. This may seem like a self-evident point, but many make choices that will in fact bring them pain. For example, they ask for what someone else has; they ask, in guidance, to influence another in their favor; and thus either they do not achieve satisfaction from the answers they get in seeking guidance, or they receive no answer at all.

The most precious things in the entire world are within you. Within you are precious stones and jewels in the form of new creative ideas, inventions, discoveries, glorious music, new songs, and answers to all problems. *The kingdom of God is within you.* (Luke 17: 21) Believe now that the subjective wisdom of your subconscious mind will direct and guide you to the right opportunity. Accept the fact of guidance now, and the door will open up. Life created you for a purpose, and you must accept your role in life. Believe that you are receiving guidance now, and you shall receive. When praying for guidance, remember that what you are seeking is always seeking you. This will give you confidence in knowing that there is an answer awaiting you.

THEY ACCEPTED GUIDANCE

At a marriage ceremony I was to perform, the bridegroom did not appear. At the end of two hours, the bride-to-be shed a few tears and then said to me, "I prayed for Divine Guidance. This might be the answer, for He never faileth."

That was her reaction—faith in God and all things good. She had no bitterness in her heart because, as she said, "It must not have been right action, because my prayer was for right action for both of us." Someone else having a similar experience would have gone into a tantrum, had an emotional fit, suffered depression, required sedation, and perhaps needed hospitalization, but this young woman accepted the guidance Divine Wisdom gave her.

※

I once lost a valuable ring that was an heirloom. I looked everywhere for it and could not locate it. At night I talked to the subconscious in the same manner that I would talk to anyone. I said to it prior to dropping off to sleep, "You know all things; you know where that ring is, and you now reveal to me where it is."

In the morning I awoke suddenly with the words ringing in my ear, "Ask Robert!"

I thought it very strange that I should ask Robert, a young boy about nine years of age; however, I followed the inner voice of guidance.

Robert said, "Oh, yes, I picked it up in the yard while I was playing with the boys. I placed it on the desk in my room. I did not think it worth anything, so I did not say anything about it."

The subconscious mind will always answer you if you trust it.

■

Alan F., a professor at a local university, attended my public lectures. After one such lecture, we started talking. I remarked that he seemed perturbed and asked him if something was wrong.

"Indeed there is," he said. "I am currently drafting a paper about archaeological excavations in Egypt during the nineteenth century. I am very nearly finished, but there is one section I cannot verify. The only reliable source for the information is a book that was privately published in a limited edition in Cairo in 1884. I've spent countless hours trying to track down a copy of the book, and so far, I have not managed to do so. Yet without it, I do not feel confident that I can submit my article for publication."

"You're in a difficult position," I said sympathetically. "May I make a suggestion?"

"Please do," he said, eager for any advice.

"Here is what I would do in a situation like yours," I continued. "Tonight, before going to bed, I would put myself into a calm, relaxed frame of mind. As I was going to sleep, I would say to myself, silently and with total confidence, 'My subconscious knows the answer, and it gives me all the information I need.' Then I would drop off to sleep with the one word, 'answer,' in my mind."

"And you believe this would be helpful?" he asked.

"Yes, I do," I replied. "Your subconscious mind is all-wise. It knows what type of answer you need. It will answer in a dream, as an overpowering hunch, or as a feeling that you are being led on the right track. You may get a sudden flash of intuition to go to a certain place, or another person may give you the answer." Later that week, Alan called me. "It's unbelievable!" he exclaimed. "I used the technique you told me about for three nights. Then, yesterday morning, as I arrived on campus, something drew me to one of the bulletin boards. Ordinarily, I walk right past them, but I couldn't. I scanned the notices, and my eye was pulled toward one announcing a used book sale to benefit a campus organization that promotes New Age ideas. It was to take place that same day at noon, on the other side of campus."

"And you went?" I asked.

"Indeed I did," he replied. "When I walked in, I wondered what I was doing there. Tables full of trashy best-selling paperbacks, volumes of condensed books, outdated software manuals, guides to building a barbecue pit . . . you know the sort of thing you find at these affairs. But at that moment, a man arrived carrying a carton of books. I heard him tell the student in charge that his late uncle was into mystical stuff like the Pyramids, and these were some of his old books."

"I think I see where you are going," I said.

"Perhaps you do," he said. "I asked if I might look through the books, since that was a field that interested me. I opened the carton, and the second book that came to hand was precisely the rare volume I had given up hope of finding! Incidentally, several other books were of great interest, too. I gave the organization a check for twice the amount they wanted to charge for the books."

At a dinner to benefit a local charity, I found myself at the same table with Adrienne W., who ran a successful media relations firm. As we chatted, the question of decision making came up. "I have a very simple technique," Adrienne said. "You may think it is too simple, but it works very well for me." Intrigued, I asked, "What is it? Will you share it with us?" "I'd be delighted," she replied. "Whenever an important question comes up that calls for a quick decision—and that seems to be at least once every day—I go into my office, shut the door, turn off the phone, and meditate on the divine qualities I believe are within me and everyone. I find myself being transported into a mood of peace, power, and confidence." A man sitting across the table, who was listening, interjected, "I'd give a lot to get some of that into *my* daily life!" "I'm sure you can, if you try," Adrienne said. "Once I find myself in that place, I say, 'Father, thou knowest all things. Give me the idea I need for this new program,' or this problem, or whatever it is. Then I visualize having the answer, feeling it flow through my mind, complete and perfect. At that point I think, 'I accept the answer and I give thanks for it.' "

The woman sitting on the other side of her, a commodities broker, said, "But you don't really have it, do you? You're just saying that." Adrienne smiled. "My grandmother used to say, 'Well begun is half done.' Once I finish my prayer, I get busy with other matters. I put the matter out of my mind. I've found that the answer usually comes when I least expect it. It's like a flash of light in a dark room that suddenly reveals everything at once. I have to say this, too: I imagine I've made as many faulty business decisions as anyone. But not once have I been disappointed by the answers that come when I follow this procedure. Not once!"

A man wrote to me saying that he had not seen his brother in over twenty years and did not know where he was. In the meantime an estate was bequeathed to both of them, and he was eager to communicate the good news to his brother. His letter reads as follows:

> Dear Dr. Murphy:
>
> I read your book, *The Miracle of Mind Dynamics*, and was very much impressed. I kept my mind focused on Infinite Intelligence; I could not see It, but based on previous experiences I was convinced of Its reality, just as I don't see the wind but I feel its breeze upon my face.
>
> I asked this Infinite Intelligence to reveal the whereabouts of my brother and I kept repeating, "Divine guidance is mine now, and Infinite Intelligence brings us together." Last week I attended a conference in New York, and lo and behold! One of the passengers who sat next to me on the subway was my brother whom I have not seen for over twenty years!
>
> I thought you might like to use this letter for the new book you are writing. I am sure this experience will instill in others faith and confidence in the mystic Power.
>
> Signed, TL, San Francisco, California.

Techniques for Finding Guidance

Some people say that they can't get ahead because they are working in a place where there is no opportunity for advancement or where wages are set by certain standards. You can use the laws of mind, however, to advance and move forward in life in any circumstances. The secret is to form a clear mental picture of what you want to be, know that the power and wisdom of your subconscious will back you up, and persevere and be determined to be what you want to be. Have faith that your desire will become your guidance. The answer will be developed in your subconscious mind and become objectified in your experience.

You can use the Infinite Power to guide someone other than yourself, whether the other be a stranger, relative, or close friend. You can do this by remembering that the Infinite Guiding Power is omnipresent and responsive to your thought and by believing in this Infinite response. I have done this for many people with extraordinary and fascinating results.

For example, a young engineer called me on the phone one day and said, "The organization I am with is selling out to a larger firm, and I am told I am not needed in the new firm. Would you pray for Divine Guidance for me?" I told him that there was an Infinite Guiding Principle that would reveal a new door of expression for him, and all he had to do was believe that this is so.

I used the principle as follows: I pictured this engineer saying to me, "I found a wonderful position with a wonderful salary. It came to me out of the blue." I did this for about three or four minutes after he hung up the phone and then forgot all about it. I believed and expected an answer. Infinite Intelligence is all-wise, and when you pray for guidance and right action, you do not tell the Infinite its business.

The following day this young man called me and confirmed the fact that he had accepted a good offer with a new engineering firm. The offer, he said, came to him "out of the blue"!

There is but one Mind, and what I subjectively pictured and felt as true came to pass in the experience of the engineer. When you call upon the Infinite Guiding Principle, It always answers you. What you believe will take place will surely happen.

In seeking guidance, think quietly about right action. You are using the Infinite Intelligence of your subconscious to the point that it takes over and begins to dominate you. From there on, your action is controlled by a subjective wisdom that knows all and sees all. When your thought is right and your motivation is right, you will be under a subconscious compulsion to do the right thing.

※

If there is a problem you've not been able to solve, as you go to sleep at night, say to your subconscious, "Give your attention to this and reveal to me the answer." You may do this silently or audibly, whichever appeals to you. When you awaken in the morning, the answer may be on your lips. If not, realize you have turned your request over with faith and confidence, and the answer will come in Divine Order. It may come as a sudden flash to your conscious mind just exactly when you need the answer.

※

Try this procedure, which many businesspeople, scientists, and others follow during their working hours.

Go to a quiet room or place, be still, relax, and think of the Infinite Intelligence and Boundless Wisdom within you, controlling all your vital forces and governing the entire cosmos with mathematical precision and unfailing accuracy. Close your eyes and focus all your attention on receiving the answer or solution. Then gently affirm, "Answer," knowing that the Infinite Intelligence within you is responsive to your request. Think of nothing but receiving the answer to your question. Continue in this quiet, relaxed, passive state of mind for a few minutes. If you find your mind wandering, bring it back to the contemplation of the answer. If you find the answer does not come in three or four minutes, let go and go on about your business. If the thought of the problem comes to your mind thereafter, just say to yourself, "I have turned my request over and Infinite Intelligence is taking care of it."

You will discover that, with this attitude, the answer will come clearly into your conscious mind. Perhaps it will come when you are engaged in some other project or when you are preoccupied with something else, but it will come.

Affirm: I give thanks for the perfect, harmonious solution that takes place through the wisdom of my Infinite Intelligence.

Principles to Remember and Apply

❯ You are spiritually equipped to overcome and to triumph over all problems, hurdles, and difficulties in life.

❯ If you are wondering about the answer to a problem that you cannot objectively solve, turn it over to your subconscious mind prior to sleep, saying, "Give your attention to this and reveal to me the answer." Guidance may be given in a dream. If it comes that way, healing currents are also released, and in the morning you feel refreshed and rejuvenated. Guidance may also come during the day, as a feeling, an inner awareness, or an overpowering hunch. Follow the guidance you receive. It never fails.

❯ When you pray for guidance and right action, take what comes. Welcome the new idea that comes into your mind in response to your prayer. Firmly believe that your new idea can bring riches into your life.

▸ Realize that as it comes from God, it is good.

▸ Realize that every problem is Divinely outmatched. Still the wheels of your mind and claim that God has the answer and that you are one with God; therefore, you also have the answer and you will receive the Divine Solution to all problems.

▸ Remember that there is always an answer. Persevere and relax, be calm and alert, so that you will recognize the lead that comes—and then follow it, and you will find wonders happening when you pray.

▸ When your motivation is right and you have no desire to take advantage of any person, and when you are praying for Divine law and order in your life, you will receive God's guidance.

▸ There is a way out of every problem and an answer to every question. Whatever you seek in life, you must go within the innermost recesses of your mind and there claim that you now are what you long to be, that you now possess what you long to possess, and your subconscious mind will reproduce what you claim and feel to be true.

▸ You know when you have really turned your problem over to your subconscious mind, because you are at peace.

▸ The Infinite Presence and Power within your deeper mind, which created the universe and all things, knows all, sees all, and has the know-how of accomplishment.

▸ Stand up to your problem with the belief that you are receiving guidance now—that the answer is within you now. Have firm conviction in the power of God to solve your problem. Your faith in the Infinite Intelligence (God) within you will enable you to overcome all problems and bring you security in any predicament.

▶ Contemplate the happy ending, and what you contemplate, you will experience.

20 Your Unlimited Power to Attract Happiness

The happiest people are the ones who constantly bring forth and practice what is best in them.

▨

*H*appiness is a state of mind.

▨

Happiness is the harvest of a quiet mind.

▨

Many people think that happiness in this life is just not going to be for them. This is due to a feeling of inferiority or rejection. The truth is that there is no such thing as an inferior or a superior person.

*Y*e are *gods; and all of you* are *children of the most High.* (Psalm 82:6)

The Life Principle does not punish, we punish ourselves by misuse of law and by negative thinking.

Your glorious destiny is to be united with God and to experience power, wisdom, strength, and illumination. Never say, "I have to resign myself to my fate", "I must put up with this", "This is God's will and I must accept it", "I'm incurable", or "It's hopeless." If you make such statements or have the mental attitude that you are here to suffer or that God is punishing or testing you for some reason, you are placing yourself in bondage, and you are degrading your Divine destiny and rejecting your very source of power to rise to untold heights.

You have the freedom to choose happiness. This may sound extraordinarily simple, and it is. Perhaps that is why people stumble over the way to happiness; they do not see the simplicity of the key to happiness. The great things in life are simple, dynamic, and creative. They are what produce well-being and happiness.

You cannot buy happiness: Some millionaires are very happy, some are very unhappy; many people with few worldly goods are very happy, and some are very unhappy, some married people are happy, and some are very unhappy; some single people are happy, and some are very unhappy.

The kingdom of happiness is in your thought and feeling.

The great deception is to enthrone the idea in your mind that things, conditions, and phenomena are the determining causes of your misery, suffering, and misfortune.

*F*or as he thinketh in his heart, so is he.
(Proverbs 23:7)

Remember, the Infinite Presence is within you. When you believe God to be punitive, therefore, you actually become your own tormentor and bring failure, lack, and misfortune onto yourself. *For they have sown the wind, and they shall reap the whirlwind.* (Hosea 8:7)

In trying to find happiness, peace, and prosperity outside of ourselves, we have neglected to look for the True Source of Happiness within ourselves, to the infinite storehouse of riches within that is our subconscious mind.

There is no block to your happiness. External things are not causative, they are effects. Your thought is your only cause, and a new cause produces a new effect.

The Life Principle moves constructively, harmoniously, rhythmically, and joyously. When we go against the principle of harmony and love or think and act in any way contrary to the forward tendency of Life, we inflict suffering upon ourselves.

Your retribution and reward depend on how you use your mind. If you make an erroneous decision in your mind, you invoke the mathematical and just response of the law of your subconscious mind, the law of action and reaction: You will experience loss as a result of your erroneous judgment or decision.

Good and evil, then, are in the movement of our minds. They are in the way we think and act and in the attitude we take toward things, not in the things themselves. The wind that blows a ship on the rocks will also bring it to a port of safety.

True and lasting happiness will come into your life the day you get the clear realization that you can overcome any weakness; that you have dominion over your thoughts; and that you realize that your subconscious can solve your problems, heal your body, and prosper you beyond your fondest dream.

You have perhaps felt the happiness of meeting your ideal mate or at the birth of your child. However, no matter how marvelous these experiences are, they do not give real lasting happiness.

The Book of Proverbs gives the answer: *Whose trusteth in the Lord, happy is he.* When you trust in the Lord (the power and wisdom of your subconscious mind) to lead, guide, govern, and direct all your ways, you will become poised, serene, and relaxed.

Many people say "If I were X, I would be happy," or "If I had X, I would be happy."

Happiness, however, consists not in acquiring material possessions whose worth to you is then so often fleeting. Happiness consists in discovering the principles of Divine Order and right action within your subconscious mind and applying these principles in all phases of your life.

There are those who see the troubles in their lives as their karma. From the standpoint of Hinduism and Buddhism, karma means action—*ka* means *to do, make,* and *ma* is *action of, result of*—and is understood as bringing upon oneself inevitable results, either good or bad, either in this life or in a reincarnation. In theory, it is the cosmic principle according to which each person is rewarded or punished in one incarnation according to his or her deeds in a previous incarnation.

Karma, however—or reaping what you have sown—is inexorable only as long as you do not pray or meditate on the truths of God. As soon as you pray, you rise above karma, and the unpleasant consequences of past mistakes begin to be wiped out. Perfunctory prayer, however, will not change matters. A deep hunger and thirst for God's love and grace, plus an intense desire to transform, are essential to wipe out the punishment that must otherwise follow negative and destructive thinking.

Epictetus, the Greek stoic philosopher, said, "There is but one way to tranquillity of mind and happiness; let this, therefore, be always ready at hand with thee, both when thou wakest early in the morning, and all the day long, and when thou goest late to sleep—to account no external things thine own, but commit all these to God."

Remember, your subconscious mind cannot act if your mind is divided. You cannot find happiness if you are harboring thoughts of doubt that lasting happiness will never be yours.

There is no block to your happiness save in your own thought-life and mental imagery.

If you misuse *any* law, you will get hurt. If you are experiencing negative reactions in life, it is not life, or your subconscious, or God being vengeful; it is simply the law of action and reaction, which is not singling you out, but which is universal and present throughout nature.

You are not a victim of the past. You can change the present, and your future will then become your present conviction made manifest—and a new beginning will become a new end.

God, the living Intelligence within you, is timeless and space-less. It is *your thoughts*, dwelling on previous actions or speech, that make you feel haunted and doomed by the past.

SHYING AWAY FROM HAPPINESS

There is one very important point about being happy: You must sincerely *desire* to be happy. Sadly, though, many people choose unhappiness. I knew a woman in England who had rheumatism for many years. She would pat herself on the knee and say, "My rheumatism is bad today. I cannot go out. My rheumatism keeps me miserable." This dear elderly lady got a lot of attention from her son, daughter, and the neighbors. She really wanted her rheumatism. She enjoyed her "misery," as she called it. This woman did not really want to be happy.

I read a newspaper article some years ago that told about a horse who had shied when he came to a stump on the road. Subsequently, every time the horse came to that same stump, he shied. The farmer dug the stump out, burned it, and leveled the old road. Yet for twenty-five years, every time the horse passed the place where the former stump was, he shied. The horse was shying at the memory of a stump.

In a like manner, you will find yourself always short of happiness if in your mind you are shying away from it—consciously or unconsciously—with doubts and fears.

A Technique for Obtaining Happiness

In the following words, Saint Paul reveals to you how you can obtain lasting happiness: *Finally; brethren, whatsoever things are true, whatsoever things are honest, whatsoever things are just, whatsoever things are pure, whatsoever things are lovely, whatsoever things are of good report; if there be any virtue, and if there be any praise, think these things.* (Philippians 4:8)

Principles to Remember and Apply

▶ There is tremendous power within you. Happiness will come to you when you acquire a sublime confidence in this power.

▶ You can rise victorious over any defeat and find happiness through the marvelous power of your subconscious mind. This is the meaning of *Whose trusteth in the Lord* [spiritual laws of the subconscious mind], *happy is he.* (Proverbs 16:20)

▶ Happiness is a habit. Choose happiness.

▶ To be happy, you must sincerely *desire* to be happy.

▶ Do not believe in things to harm or hurt you. Believe in the power of your subconscious to heal, inspire, strengthen, and prosper you. According to your belief is it done unto you.

▶ You cannot buy happiness. The kingdom of happiness is in your thought and feeling.

▶ Happiness is the harvest of a quiet mind. Anchor your thoughts in peace.

> The happiest people are the ones who bring forth the highest and the best in themselves.

> Your joy and suffering are the reflections of your habitual thinking.

Epilogue

WORLD PEACE

You and I are the ones to initiate peace by changing our minds and hearts.

Once, when I was giving a series of lectures in Palm Springs, a man in the hotel where I was staying asked me to sign a paper outlawing war. He said that he had 20,000 signatures so far and that he expected to obtain millions of signatures, then he was going to submit them to Congress and insist that they pass a law outlawing war and influence other nations to do the same. All this is so much balderdash and folderol.

In our conversation, I explained to him that men could sign all the documents for peace in every parliament in the world, and it would be of no avail. History shows and proves that many governmental decrees and formal agreements and pledges for peace have been signed by numerous nations but, often before the ink wherewith they were written could dry, they were broken. Parliaments and legislatures of the world cannot legislate peace, harmony, security, abundance or love of neighbor—all these are ordained and legislated in the minds and hearts of man. Peace begins with the individual, and if a man has peace within himself he will be at peace with his wife, his friends and associates, as well as with all the world.

War is caused by fear, hate, greed, revenge, anger, and the lust of men. If a man is full of anger, resentment, hostility, and suppressed rage, he is at war with himself and his world.

A nation is an aggregation of individuals; therefore, the only place to write legislation for peace is by the individual tuning in on the God of peace within himself and feeling that river of peace, love, harmony, and joy flowing through him. Furthermore, when man realizes that he can go to the Infinite Mind within himself and there claim and feel what he wants to be, to do, and to have, the Infinite Intelligence will respond accordingly, and he will discover that he can have what he wants without hurting the hair of a living being.

Another question raised at one of my lectures was "If God is love and if He is All-Good and All-Wise, why doesn't He stop war, crime, murder, and rape? Why does He permit thousands and millions of children to die of hunger and countless other thousands to become crippled and maimed by the ravages of war?"

The answer is that God—the Universal Being, the Cosmic Power, the Supreme and Infinite Intelligence—works on a cosmic scale or from the standpoint of the Universal. In other words, God is Presence in the Cosmic plane, moving as unity, harmony, rhythm, order, beauty, and proportion.

The law, simply stated, however, is that the Universal can only act on the plane of the particular or individual by *becoming* the individual. The only way God can work *for* us is *through* you— through our thoughts, feelings, and mental imagery.

God can't stop wars, crime, disease, discord, and accidents.

You and I are the ones to initiate peace by changing our minds and hearts. Then, as we think in our hearts, it will be done unto us. Our world will be at peace.

There is no one to change but yourself.

Start now.

Printed in the United States
by Baker & Taylor Publisher Services